THE CORE OF THE MATTER

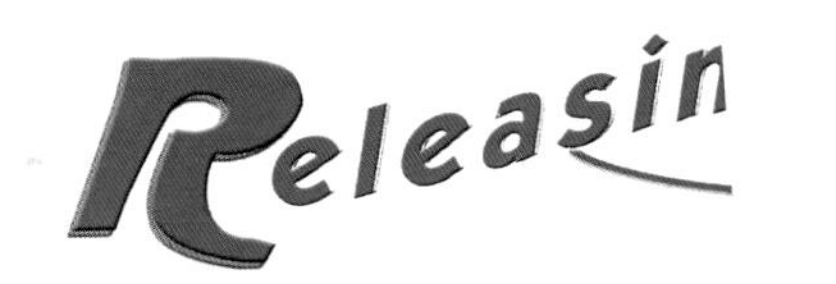

THE ILIOPSOAS AND QUADRATUS LUMBORUM

Restoring power, ease, and fluidity to the low back and pelvis

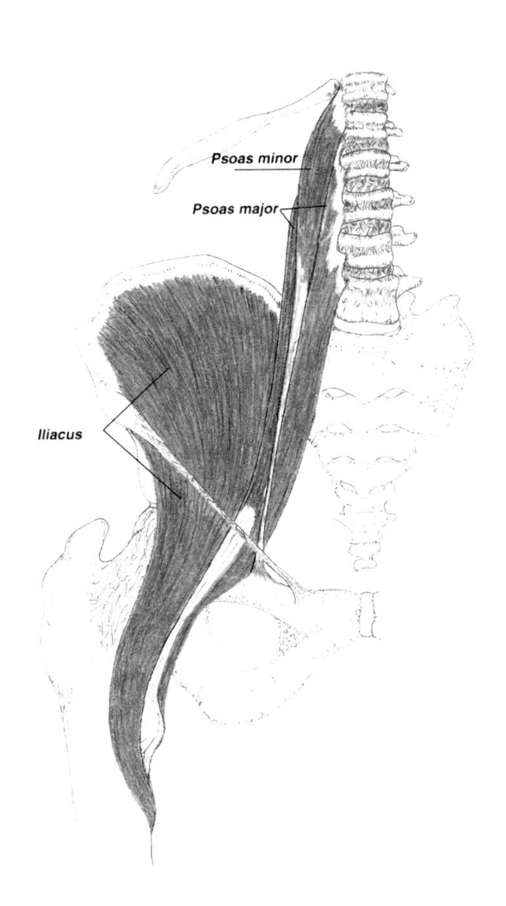

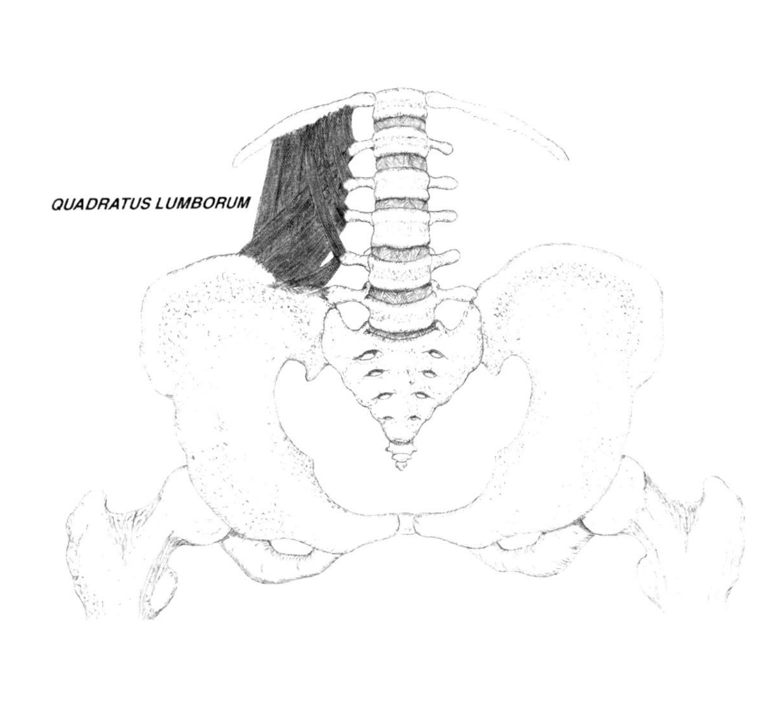

Peggy Lamb, MA, LMT, NCTMB

Dedication

To Jerre Yarbrough (1933 - 2011) beloved mentor, teacher, and friend.

She burned her presence into me
My psyche, my cells, my soul
The wind blew through her
As she hissed her hands into my body
Digging, pressing, kneading
The core of my being
A stream of flame burst out of her fingers
She lit the fire in my belly
A birthing of Womanhood
She was my labor coach
Rocking me, petting me, pushing me
Through sorrow and rage
Into power

Disclaimer:
Low back and hip/pelvic problems can be complex, multidimensional and multifaceted. This book is not a comprehensive study of those issues. This manual is for educational purposes only and should not be considered a substitute for proper training. It is sold with the understanding that the author and publisher are not engaged in rendering medical or other professional services. If medical advice or other expert assistance is required, the services of an appropriate professional should be sought. Information in this book should not be used to diagnose, treat, or prescribe. The author and publisher shall not be held liable for any damages in connection with, or arising out of anyone's interpretation or application of the information in this manual. The practitioner is encouraged to always use sound clinical judgment in making decisions about her/his ability to help each individual and to refer to a qualified professional when the need arises.

Photographs by Carol Waid and Peg Runnels
Illustrations by Diana Ross
With deep gratitude to MaryAnn Reynolds for her expert editing, my models, Tracy Firsching and Lela Reynolds for their patience with multiple takes and Frank Kroncke and Tracy Firsching for their insights and edits.

Additional copies of this book may be obtained from:

www.massagepublications.com

or

Massage Publications
8400 Jamestown Dr #118
Austin, TX 78758

(512) 833-0179

or email

info@massagepublications.com

Table of Contents

A TALE OF TWO MUSCLES

Our appendicular skeleton, in large part, determines how we communicate and move through life. The quality of our communication and the vitality of our movement are directly determined by the health and flexibility of our axial skeleton/core.

The two principal muscles in this book, the iliopsoas and quadratus lumborum, are prime time players in determining whether we are free to move through life with power, ease and fluidity. They are like the mother and father in a stable and functional family where the children (the arms and legs) can go out into the world freely, returning home again and again to a stable center.

Although this book focuses on low back/hip pain, these muscles play a much more complex role in determining our overall health. I focus on these two muscles because, as a teacher of bodywork, I have long observed that many of my students are unsure and wary of working them, especially the dreaded iliopsoas.

If you've ever had the heebie-jeebies and shirked away from palpating and releasing the iliopsoas, this book is for you. It will enable you to increase your skills by learning how to precisely palpate the iliopsoas and quadratus lumborum. Or, if the techniques you've learned for releasing these formidable muscles are akin to some Spanish Inquisition practices, you'll discover gentle, effective, and safe protocols for restoring health to these muscles by using my *Muscle Swimming* technique, which has the added benefit of saving your hands. By using the information and techniques presented in this book, you'll be able to restore biomechanical integrity and create normal length-tension relationships in these muscles and others while respecting and honoring your own ecology of movement and effort.

Since low back pain is the second most common reason for patient visits to the doctor's office[1], second only to upper repository infections, understanding the role these two extraordinary muscles play in low back health is of vital importance to any bodyworker using manual therapy to relieve client's low back pain.

My fascination with these muscles comes from personal experience. As a dancer in graduate school I developed rigid patterns of movement while diligently (and unsuccessfully) striving to have perfect technique. The protocols presented in this book are sourced in my twenty-five plus years of being a bodyworker. Many have arisen as part of my own healing journeys with my problematic and cantankerous hips.

1 American Chiropractic Association

THE CORE OF THE MATTER

The iliopsoas—a complicated, multifaceted, multitasking, passion vine of a muscle—winds its way from front to back, inside to outside, and top to bottom. It is a conduit and messenger between our legs (attachment at the lesser trochanter) pelvis,upper body and even our arms (attachment at T12). One of my early teachers said that having his iliopsoas released was a mystical experience. I agree wholeheartedly. I fervently believe that if we work *with* the iliopsoas—as opposed to working *on* it or on any other muscle—that the work can be a powerful and liberating experience for clients as well as therapists.

The quadratus lumborum is the infamous "crawl to the bathroom" muscle (the low back pain is so intense that walking to the bathroom is impossible) because it contributes so powerfully to core stabilization. It is a stalwart, thick bodied and protective muscle that creates and maintains a profound and primal stability. It is a deeply rooted, sturdy shrub—or if it was an animal, a bear. When it gets angry, it roars and the stable house often comes tumbling down. Like the iliopsoas, it connects the upper body to the lower body via the ilium, but it doesn't have the long, vine-like reach of the psoas. It is short and squat like a shrub with its branches (fibers) going off in different directions to their bony attachments. The complexity of the quadratus lumborum's fiber arrangement—some vertical, some diagonal in one direction, some diagonal in the other direction—is what makes this muscle so strong and steady. Of course, if these fibers lose their way and get twisted and tangled, which frequently happens, the quadratus lumborum can wreak havoc in our lives.

MUSCLE SWIMMING

Do your hands and body hurt after working with clients? You are not alone. It's time for all bodyworkers to work smarter, not harder with minimum effort and maximum results. Since every muscle has an automatic sensory reflex whose job it is to resist sudden change from external forces, let's retire Atilla the Thumb and go *Muscle Swimming* instead.

Simply put, Muscle Swimming means incorporating active and passive movement while you work with the tissue. Active and passive movement strategies are an essential ingredient in all the protocols in this book. Movement allows our fingers to swim and sink into the tissue. The powerful combination of active and passive movement maneuvers turns off hyperactivity in muscles and joint receptors. It also facilitates the separation and lifting of fascial layers. With each *active* movement we "take it to the brain" involving our wondrous central nervous system and neurology.

The two primary techniques of Muscle Swimming are *Pin and Rock* and *Pin and Move.* Pin and Rock is a powerful strategy that serves as a portal to deep tissue work. The therapist gradually presses to find the tissue's first barrier. Then the muscle is gently pinned, and the therapist adds slow rocking. Rocking has an immediate calming effect. It stimulates the parasympathetic system, harking us back to the time when we were rocked for nine months in the womb. Think of it as a way of introducing yourself and saying hello to the tissue.

Pin and Move is an effective and intelligent strategy to work through myofascial layers after warming the tissue with *Pin and Rock.* The therapist pins a stubborn trigger point or tender area while the client performs active movement.

Giving your client specific movement instructions and encouraging them to move intuitively during the session grants your client ownership of the important and sacred process of realigning and reclaiming her core.

EMOTIONAL MUSCLES

I've included body/mind considerations and thoughts for each muscle. I am not advocating violating our scope of practice and becoming armchair psychotherapists. For me—and I hope for you—when I touch a muscle I believe that I am touching the whole person—emotions, thoughts, energies and soul.

Consider letting my beliefs about the emotions/energies associated with our beautiful friends, the iliopsoas and quadratus lumborum, float in the back of your body/mind as you work with your clients. Consider offering support and guidance from your intuition, without psychoanalyzing anyone.

For example, if you sense that a client's chronic problems with her quadratus lumborum might be associated with feeling unsupported, you can gently suggest that she lie on the floor and soak in the deep sensation of being supported by our stable and strong Mother Earth. Or, for the iliopsoas, perhaps blocked energy in the pelvis might be dissipated by imitating the swirling of a hula-hoop. These kinds of suggestions are appropriate if offered from a non-judgmental place of compassionate detachment.

I strongly recommend that every therapist receives work on these muscles before working on the iliopsoas and quadratus lumborum with clients. Personally, receiving deep and profound work provided me with the foundation to intuitively work on others. I knew much about what my clients were experiencing, and those self-insights gave me the confidence to experiment and boldly (although not aggressively) go with my clients into uncharted territory.

IN CONCLUSION

There are numerous ways to approach these muscles. Being skilled in a wide variety of therapeutic interventions allows us to serve our clients with excellence. Finally, let us always remember that no matter how good we get technically, *"We do not bless with our expertise, we bless with our bare hands."* (Said by the magnificent and wise writer Rachel Remen, MD at the WomenSpeak Conference 2007.)

Principles of Muscle Swimming

As manual therapists we all face the question, "How can I best facilitate tissue release and allow the muscle to return to its happy, healthy resting state while maintaining my own ecology of movement?" I stumbled across an answer to that dilemma about twelve years ago and have been refining my approach ever since in both my private practice and seminars. Simply put, Muscle Swimming uses physiology to facilitate release of myofascial structures allowing the therapist to work smarter and the client to have co-ownership of the session. The following are the core components of Muscle Swimming:

1. Warm the tissue with Swedish strokes before deep tissue work.

2. *Pin and Rock:* our first encounter with a stressed myofascial unit should be gentle and non-threatening. Passively shorten the muscle, gently pin it with multiple fingers for a broad, dispersed pressure and add a slow rhythmic rocking of the joint. Rocking stimulates a parasympathetic response. After all, we are rocked for nine months. In fact, the first nerves to myelinate in the human fetus are the vestibular nerves which sense movement. Our first consciousness is that we are a moving beings. Be patient – wait for the tissue to soften and yield before moving to the Pin and Move protocol. Come back to this Pin and Rock maneuver whenever you sense guarding in your client.

3. *Pin and Move:* when you meet an area of dense fascia, trigger points, tender points or just plain snarly tissue, integrate active movement. Active movement "takes it to the brain", involving the central nervous system, creating longer lasting results. Fascial layers and actin and myosin myofibrils glide across each other as the muscle goes through its shortened, neutral and stretched states.

A. Place the muscle in a shortened state.

B. Pin the area at first barrier. If it's a trigger point or tender point, use one finger, or appropriate tool for specificity and work it from an oblique angle of 45 degrees.

C. Have your client do a movement. Start with the main action the muscle performs, i.e. flexion, abduction, extension etc. Movement should be done at a slow to medium tempo.

D. Client repeats the movement 4-5 times.

E. Ask your client if the area or point is better, worse or the same. If your client says that the area is better, your nest question is, "how much better?" If your client reports at least a 50% change for the better, then move to another area and repeat the above steps.

F. If your client reports no change you have three options:

1. Add resistance to the current movement pattern. This loads the muscle and recruits more fibers, allowing you to swim through the tissue. 10 - 20% of resistance is usually all that is needed. For example, your client is performing thigh flexions while you pin a stubborn trigger point in the iliopsoas. To add resistance, simply place your downhill hand on the thigh, add 10 - 20% of resistance and ask your client to

continue the thigh flexions.

2. Try another movement pattern. Adding resistance to the new pattern is always an option.

3. Ask your client for input. She may feel an itch to move the joint in a certain way.

G. If your client reports that the point or area is worse that is not necessarily a negative outcome. It's possible that through the portal of Active Movement, you've swum to a trigger point or congested area at a deeper layer of tissue. The same three options apply to this situation as well:

1. Add resistance to the current movement pattern.

2. Try another movement pattern. Adding resistance to the new pattern is always an option.

3. Ask your client for input. She may feel an itch to move the joint in a certain way.

4. Work the muscle(s) from as many different positions as possible — supine, side-lying, prone, and even weight-bearing. Perhaps your client is a golfer suffering from low back pain and the quadratus lumborum is the main culprit. Have him go through a golf swing while you work the tissue. Think outside the box and get the client moving!

5. When you find an exquisitely tender spot or trigger point, work to release the tissue around it before concentrating on the tender point.

6. Give your client a break! Working on these muscles, especially the iliopsoas, can be quite stressful. Incorporate what I call the "sweet stuff" during your deep tissue work, i.e., energy work, a short foot massage, some relaxing effleurage, etc.

7. Breath connects us all! Breathe deeply while working and encourage your client to do the same.

8. Combine working two muscles at the same time. Since all muscles work interdependently this is an especially effective release technique.

9. Practice patience, non-judgment, curiosity, and compassion.

10. If it hurts you, don't do it! Adapt the technique to suit your body.

Contraindications for Muscle Swimming:

1. Infection
2. Non-united fracture or scar
3. Open wound
4. Hematoma
5. Sutures
6. Any condition for which movement would be harmful to the client. Obtain medical clearance first. When in doubt, leave it out!

If your client does not show significant improvement in 4-6 sessions, refer to a doctor.

The following pages present techniques and protocols for releasing the iliopsoas and quadratus lumborum. These techniques and protocols are *"a way"* not *"the way"* and are there to serve as guidelines or trail markers. The muscles do not have to be worked in the order presented. It's practical to do all your supine or prone work at the same time.

Each client is unique and presents us with creative challenges in the use of our skills, intuition, and knowledge. Expand and enlarge upon the following techniques and protocols with your knowledge and creativity. Know the actions and attachments of the muscle you are working. A strong foundational knowledge of anatomy is indispensable for intelligent, intuitive bodywork. It allows you to know where you are going as you follow your fingers.

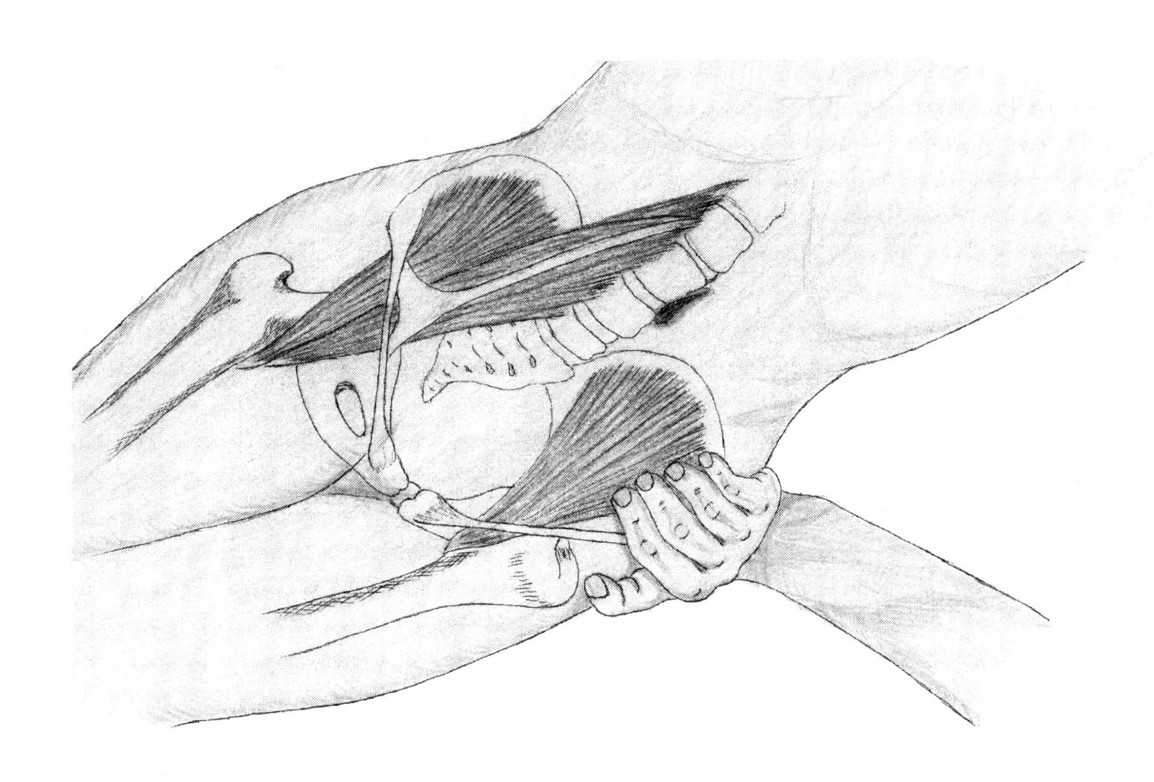

ILIOPSOAS

Attachments: *Psoas* — (above) 12th thoracic vertebrae and all lumbar vertebrae and corresponding discs; (below) lesser trochanter of the femur. *Iliacus* — (above) upper two-thirds of the inner surface of the iliac fossa, anchoring to the lip of the iliac crest completely lining the wall of the pelvis; (below) most of the iliacus fibers join with the psoas to attach to the lesser trochanter.
Actions: flexion of the thigh at the hip; flexion of the torso; plays a significant role maintaining upright posture. Eccentrically, the iliopsoas check-reins hyperextension of the thigh.

The temperamental, or as Tom Myers called it, the opinionated iliopsoas, is one of the major muscle complexes of the body. This long sausage of a muscle is involved with the entire working mechanics of the back, pelvis, legs, and indirectly, the arms. It initiates walking and serves as a major postural stabilizer by contributing to the natural curve of the lumbar spine by controlling the pelvic tilt. An unhappy, irate iliopsoas can cause a kinetic chain reaction up to the neck and down to the big toe. Quite often it is the hidden culprit in stubborn low back pain.

The iliopsoas connects via fascia to the diaphragm, providing root support. Releasing the T12 attachment of the psoas often results in deeper and full-bodied breathing. The rhythmic waves produced from a fully engaged diaphragm can assist in restoring core stability and spinal flexibility.

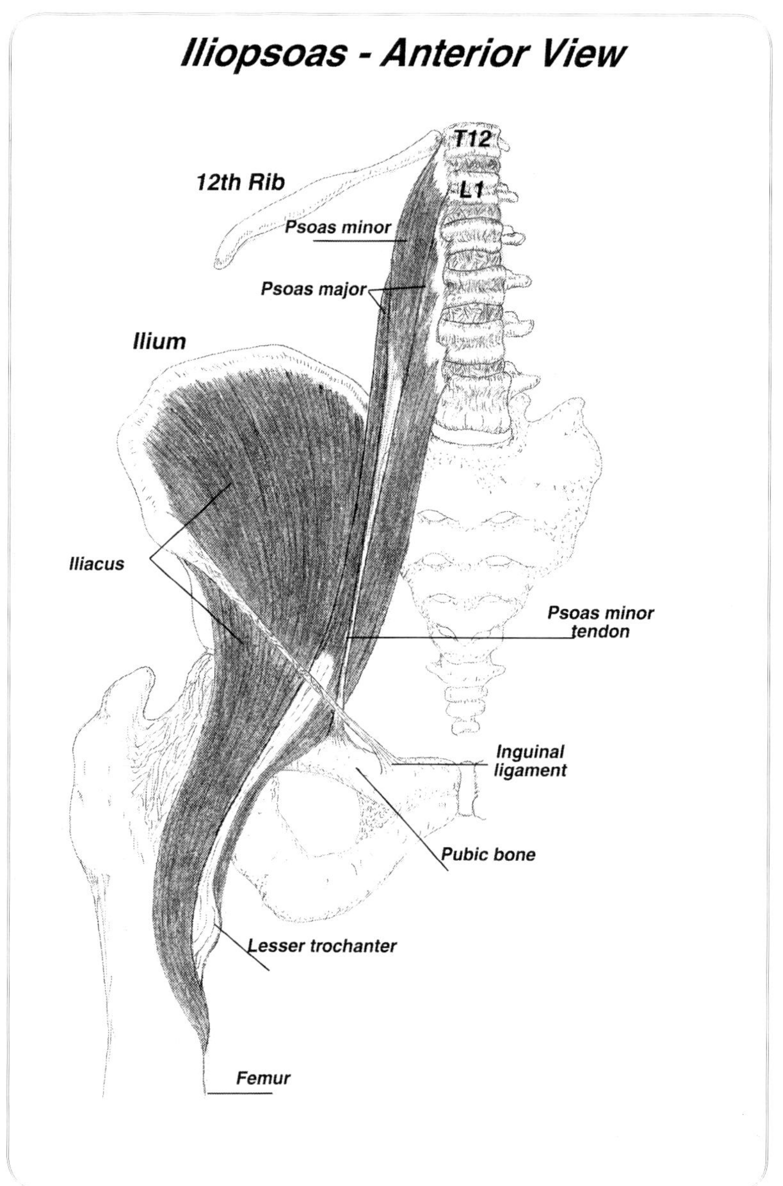

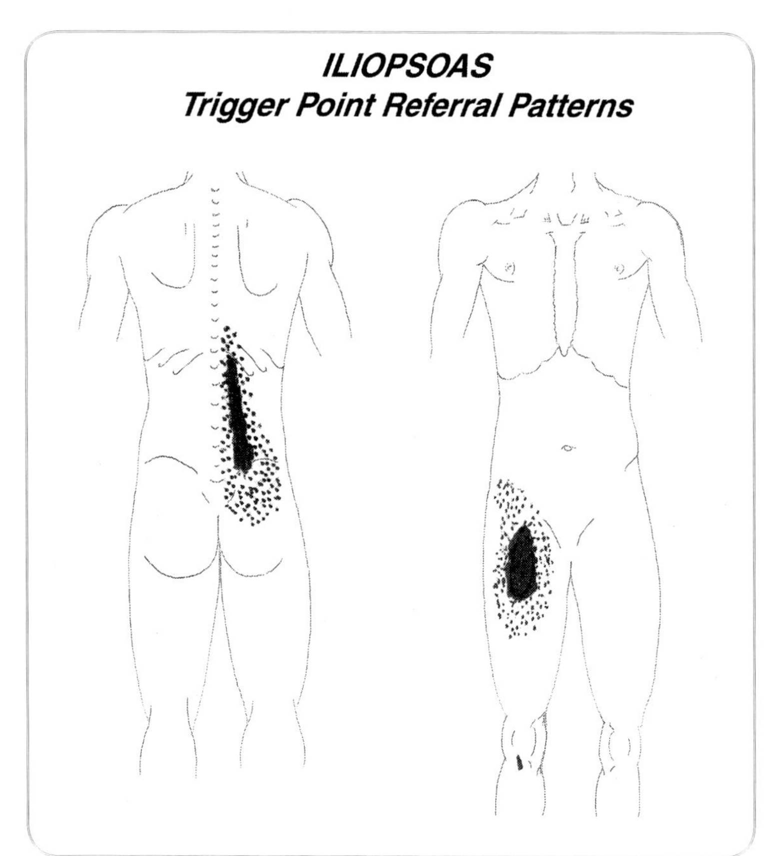

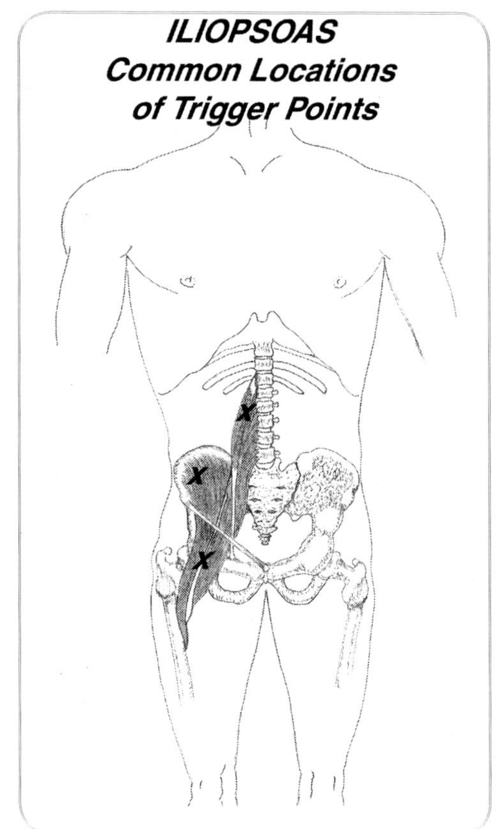

Trigger points refer in a vertical pattern ipsilaterally (same side) on the lumbar spine, the anterior thigh, and sometimes the patella tendon just below the knee. Activation of trigger points/dysfunction of the iliopsoas is multi-dimensional. A few common causes are: prolonged sitting with the hips in the jack-knifed position, sleeping in the fetal position with the knees drawn up to the chest, tightness of the rectus femoris muscle that prevents full hip extension, and—last but certainly not least—weak and/or incorrectly trained abdominal muscles. (See Client Education section for suggestions on how to properly train the abdominals.)

Sacroiliac instability contributes to overtaxing the iliopsoas, and its robust partner in core stability, the quadratus lumborum. When sacral, lumbar, and pelvic ligaments weaken or when the pelvic bowl is off center, guess who gets called on to pick up the slack? The iliopsoas, leaving it overburdened and exhausted and unable to contribute to thigh flexion as much as it should. In turn, the secondary hip flexors, (tensor fascia latae, sartorius, pectineus and rectus femoris, adductors longus, brevis, and magnus) get overwhelmed, wondering where the heck is that iliopsoas? In fact, I've often found on myself and others that it is these smaller, synergistic, helper muscles that send off the first obnoxious pain signals. A sharp, grabbing pain at the front of the hip when the thigh is extended, such as standing after sitting or getting in and out of a car, is a common complaint. Since many people spend the day sitting, the thigh flexors are often left in a shortened state, increasing the anterior pelvic tilt. When we stand up, the thigh and pelvis extends, which puts an eccentric demand on the thigh flexors, a demand they vociferously protest at times. These secondary thigh flexors often do not get the attention they deserve. I suggest working them before the iliopsoas.

The iliopsoas is truly multifaceted as it performs a variety of actions in addition to its critical function as a postural stabilizer. Bringing its inferior attachment (lesser trochanter) toward its superior attachment (T12) produces thigh flexion. Do the opposite and, voila, you've got trunk flexion. We can even do them both at the same time. Try it.

1. Stand on your dominant leg. Think of sending thick roots out of your foot into the earth.
2. Bring your non-dominant thigh towards your belly (thigh flexion.)
3. Keeping your spine long, move your upper body towards your thigh (trunk flexion.)
4. Upper and lower body say hello to each other.

AN EMOTIONAL MUSCLE

Alexander Lowen, MD, the brilliant creator of BioEnergetic Therapy, wrote, "There is a bottom to our despair. It is the pelvic floor." Although the iliopsoas is not technically a pelvic floor muscle, it is certainly part of the floor's fascial web. It absorbs and transmits whatever disturbances are present in the pelvic floor; it is in the same neighborhood association, so to speak.

At an early age, many of us learn to tighten the pelvic floor as a strategy of self-control. It's a common flight or fight mechanism that serves to repress frightening emotions. The iliopsoas, being a major flexor muscle, is an essential part of the fear reflex, pulling the body into a fetal position (trunk and thigh flexion) and so protecting our soft vulnerable parts.

The solar plexus, sometimes called the abdominal or "stomach brain," lies approximately at the level where psoas and diaphragm intersect. Tissue restriction here can interfere with trusting our gut feelings and instincts.

The path of the iliopsoas is through the belly of the whale where our personal demons, traumas, and wounds live, along with our dreams, visions, vitality, sexuality and creativity. Within this area is the source of our adaptability and our ability to form relationships and associations outside ourselves.

We live in a culture with strange and damaging notions about sexuality. One of the most prevalent of these cultural messages is to suck in the belly. After all, we should all strive for Barbie and Ken bodies, right? All the energy that goes into struggling for six-pack abdominals results in rigid movement patterns and restricts the natural sway of the hips. Many cultures value fluid, swaying hips and rounded bellies. Elvis Presley (Elvis the Pelvis) was shocking in his early years because he dared to move his hips with abandon and pleasure in public. Our culture hasn't become much wiser and sexually mature since then — toxic ideas about sexuality are implanted in us daily through the media.

Energetic and psychological imbalances in the iliopsoas can manifest as sexual troubles. If there's too much energy, the person may be sexually overactive; too little energy and the person may be dispassionate about sex and relationships.

The iliopsoas initiates walking, our active reaching through space. Fears about our ability to stretch for our dreams and expressing ourselves can lodge in our lovely iliopsoas.

We must approach this deep, mysterious muscle with reverence and caution. Perhaps direct mechanical intervention is not called for in all clients, especially if there is a history of sexual abuse, rape, or torture. If you find that your client glaringly tenses up and blocks your entry to the iliopsoas, honor that boundary. You can offer support by guiding them through the list of active movements found in the Movement Suggestions section. These movements are designed to restore innate proprioception to an area that may have been shut down for years.

PROTOCOLS FOR RELEASING THE ILIOPSOAS AND SECONDARY THIGH FLEXORS

In this section you'll find:

1. Assessment tests and preliminary corrections
2. Positional Release technique
3. Protocols for releasing the secondary thigh flexors
4. Protocols for releasing the iliopsoas
5. Active movement suggestions for Muscle Swimming
6. Table stretches

Contraindications for Working the Iliopsoas

1. Pregnancy
2. Women who are menstruating
3. Hernia
4. If your client has a history of trauma (abuse of any kind, rape, torture, etc.) approach this work with caution. If you do not feel comfortable bearing witness to the intense emotions that may arise, please refer to a psychotherapist or a body/mind therapist

Precautions for Working the Iliopsoas

1. Avoid pressure on the viscera by muscle testing for muscle fiber to contract.
2. Avoid pressure on neurovascular structures which lie medial to the psoas.
3. When working the iliopsoas, ask your client to let you know if she feels hot, gassy or searing pain. If she does, you've probably impinged some intestinal tissue. Simply release the tissue and use a different angle.
4. Be aware of any abdominal surgeries —avoid the area if the surgery is recent.

Assessment Tests

Assessment tests are useful guidelines that, along with postural observations, gait assessment, pain patterns, and palpation can give us a global picture to keep in mind as we work locally. I've included the following assessment tests that I perform before and after the deep tissue/trigger point and stretching protocols:

1. Test for a short iliopsoas
2. Test for pelvic tilt.
3. Preliminary corrections for pelvic tilt.
4. Also included is a simple positional release technique for a short iliopsoas. I've found that doing this easy procedure along with the preliminary corrections for pelvic tilt prepares the muscles for the deep tissue/trigger point protocols.

TEST 1: Test for short iliopsoas

Client is supine with no bolster under the knees and the knees are extended. Therapist stands at the head of the table.

Step 1: Have client bring both arms next to her ears and place her palms together, fingers extended (prayer position).

Step 2: Gently take hold of the arms just below the wrist and lean back. Make sure you have a gentle even pull on both arms.

Step 3: Place your hands over her hands and move her arms overhead. Check to see which *thumb* is shorter. The short side iliopsoas creates an inferior and contralateral rotation on the spine because of its attachment at T12. This results in one arm being slightly shorter than the other. **Work the short side first**. Always work both sides, although one side will usually require more attention.

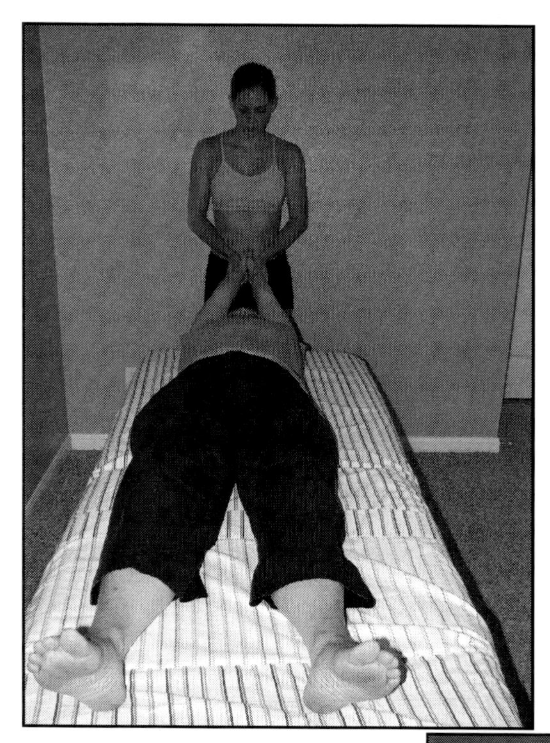

Step 1

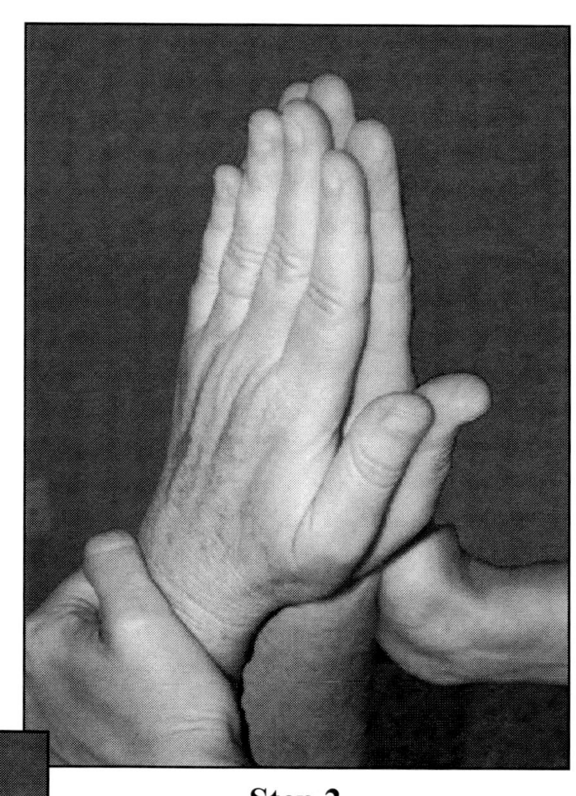

Step 2

Step 3: ***This person's left thumb is shorter***

TEST 2: Test for pelvic tilt

In this test you'll determine if your client has an anterior pelvic tilt, a posterior pelvic tilt or a normal pelvic tilt. We'll use the relationship of two bony landmarks, the anterior superior iliac spine (ASIS) and the posterior superior iliac spine (PSIS). As a general rule, the ASIS varies from directly anterior of the PSIS to 1/2 inch inferior of the PSIS. Deviations within this range are considered normal. If the ASIS is more than 1/2 inch inferior to the PSIS the client has an excessive anterior tilt. If the ASIS is superior to the PSIS the client has a posterior tilt of the pelvis. Most of your clients with low back pain will have one of these conditions.

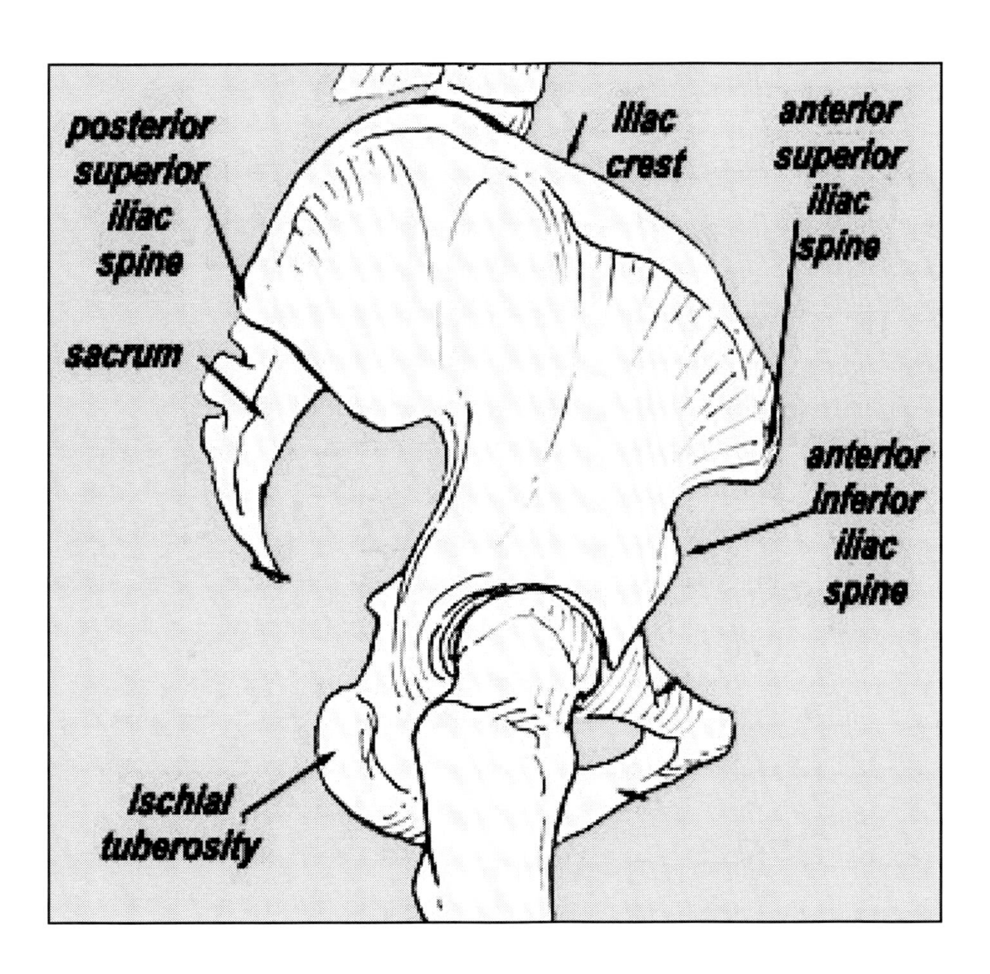

Client is standing. Kneel at the side of the client.

Step 1: Place one finger on the center of her PSIS. Find the PSIS by placing your thumbs on the posterior medial section of the pelvis. Lower your thumbs about 1/2 inch. Feel for the dimples that most people have. Just beneath these dimples, feel for a small bony protuberance. This is the PSIS. It takes a bit of practice — if you've never done it before, be bold and ask your friends and family to participate in a palpation exercise.

Step 2: Find the ASIS by placing your finger on the anterior medial portion of the iliac crest. The ASIS will be just inferior to your fingers. You may ask your client to lean forward (trunk flexion) to help find the ASIS. Hook your finger inferior to her ASIS.

Step 3: Lean back and extend your elbows.

Step 4: Test the other side.

Step 5: Record findings.

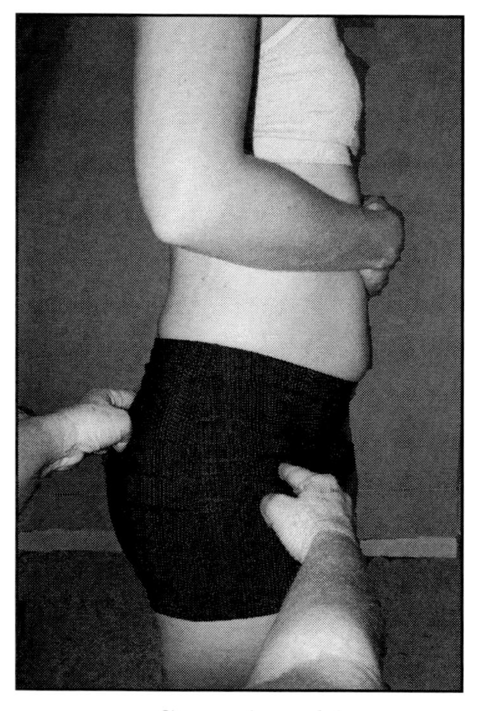

Steps 1 and 2

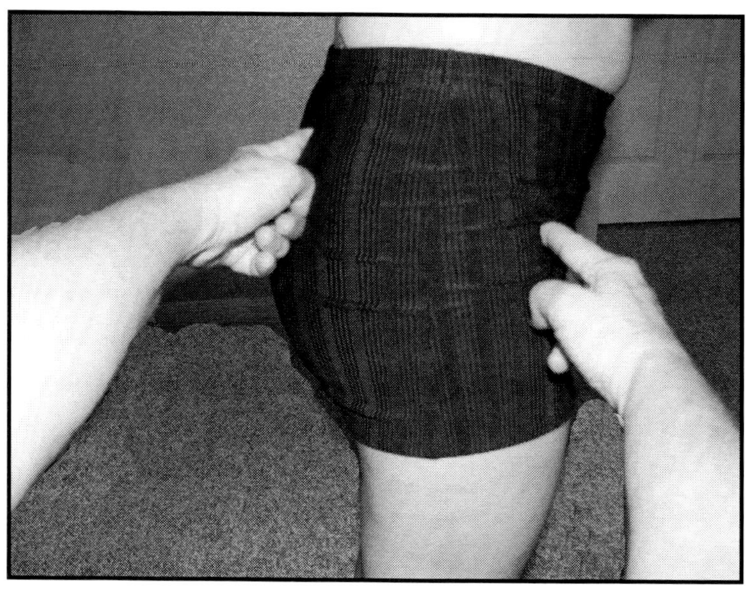

Step 3: Her ASIS is about a 1/2 inch inferior to her PSIS so her pelvic tilt is normal.

Preliminary correction for anterior pelvic tilt

Think of this maneuver as a gentle repositioning of the bones rather than a stretch.

Client is supine.

Step 1: Bend knee and flex the thigh of the excessively anteriorly tilted pelvis. If both sides are affected, do this protocol on both sides.

Step 2: Reach under the ischium and pull the back of the pelvis caudally toward the feet as you gently push the thigh to her chest as far as possible.

Step 3: Instruct client to take a deep breath, hold it, then gently (5-10% of effort) push the buttock down toward the massage table isometrically as you provide resistance by gently pushing up. Have them hold the contraction for 6-8 seconds, then relax/exhale and repeat 2-3 times. Feel for the slight yielding of the pelvis in a posterior direction.

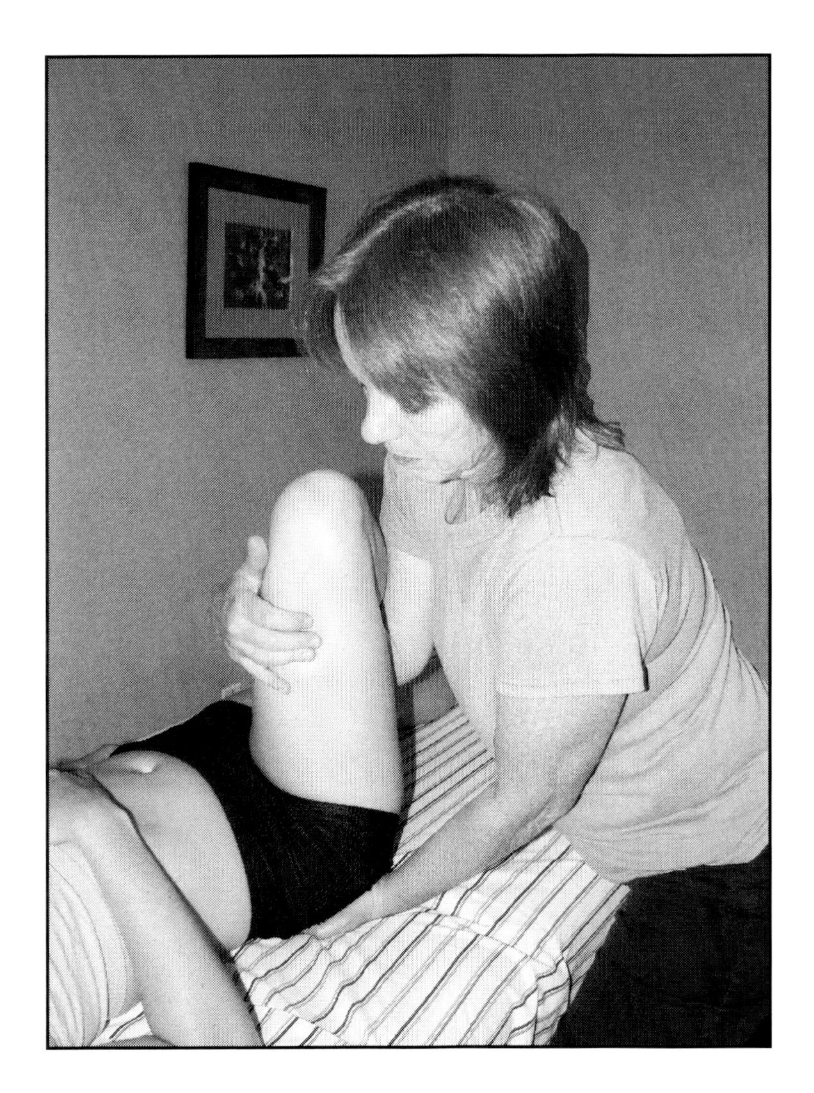

Preliminary correction for posterior pelvic tilt

Think of this maneuver as a gentle repositioning of the bones rather than a stretch.

Client is side-lying on the opposite side of the posteriorly tilted pelvis. If both sides are affected, do this protocol on both sides.

Step 1: Ask your client to bend her knee and flex the thigh of the bottom leg to stabilize the pelvis.

Step 2: Hyperextend the top leg back as far as comfortably possible to encourage a re-positioning of the pelvis. You may wrap the leg around your waist to help hold the weight of the leg. Your uphill hand should be pushing the ischium up toward the head to prevent the low back from an uncomfortable lordosis as your other hand pulls the top leg back into hyperextension.

Step 3: Instruct client to take a deep breath, hold it and gently (5-10% of effort) flex the thigh isometrically as you provide resistance. Have her hold the contraction for 6-8 seconds, then relax/exhale and repeat 2-3 times. Feel for the slight yielding of the pelvis in an anterior direction.

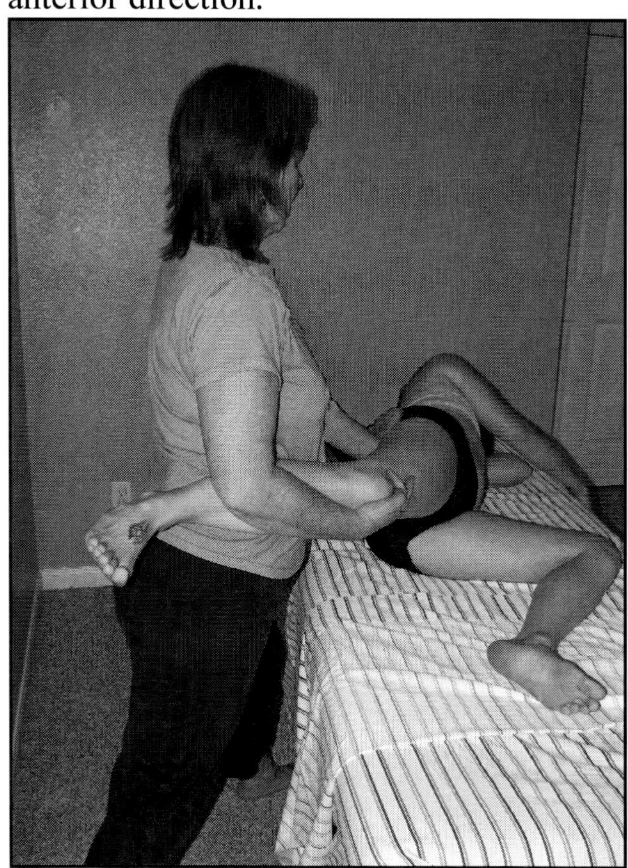

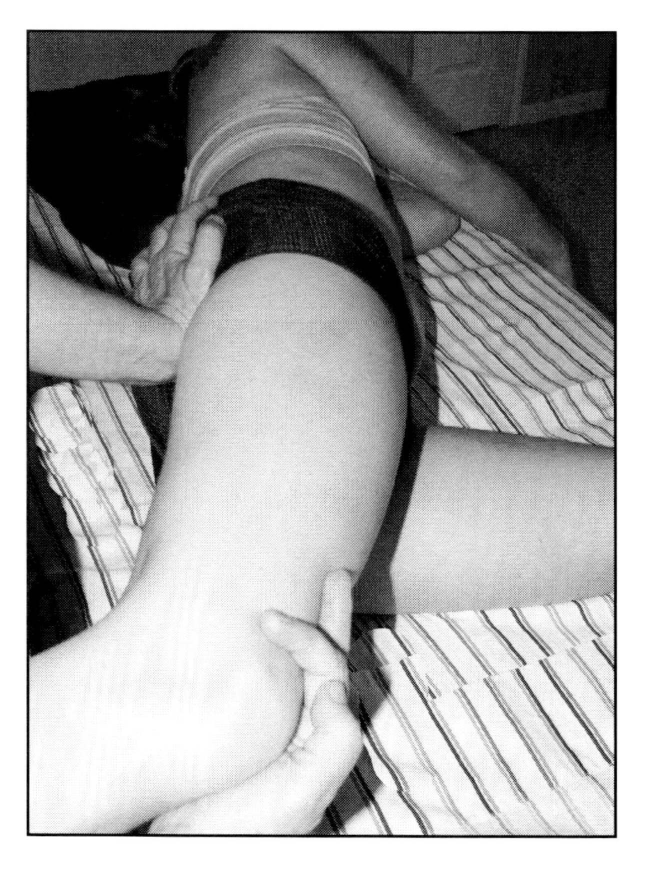

POSITIONAL RELEASE FOR SHORT ILIOPSOAS

This is an excellent "pre-release" of the iliopsoas that prepares the muscle and the client for deeper work directly on the muscle. I find it to be valuable in creating receptivity in the tissue. The technique is simply to place the muscle in a passive shortened state and hold about two minutes.

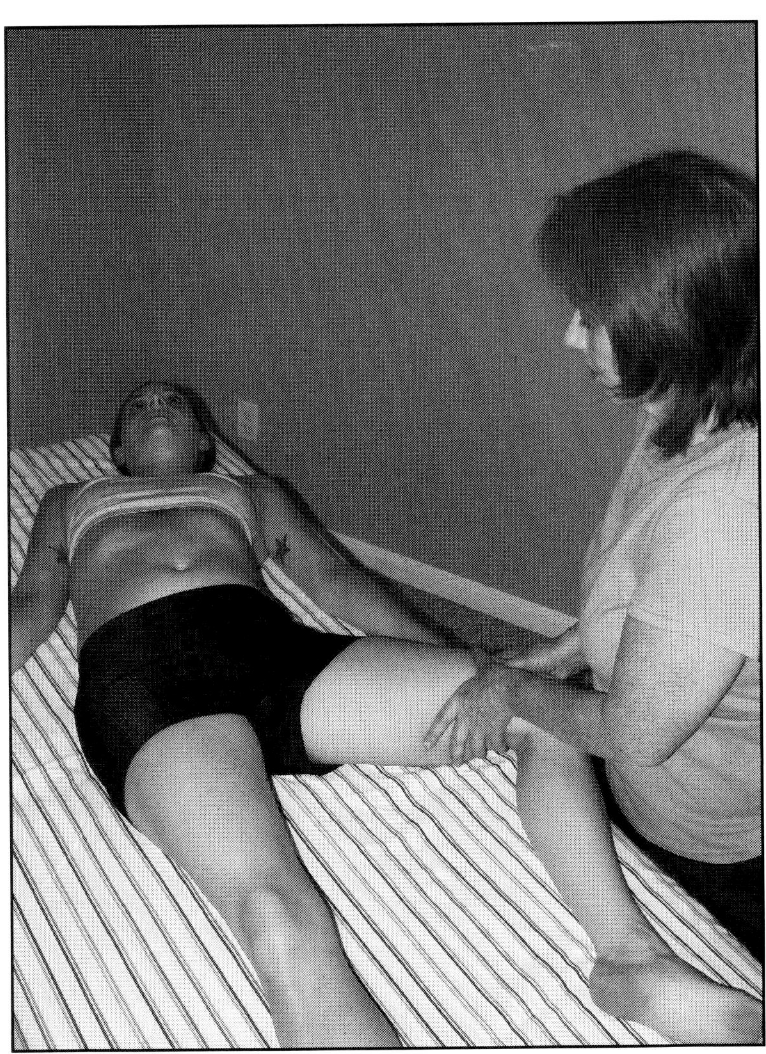

Client is supine.

Step 1: Side bend the torso on the affected (short) side.

Step 2: Externally rotate and slightly abduct the thigh.

Step 3: Gently compress (push) the femur up into the hip joint with your hands.

Step 4: Hold for about two minutes.

Protocols for Releasing the Secondary Thigh Flexors

We begin our deep tissue work with the secondary thigh flexors *(tensor fascia latae, sartorius, pectineus and rectus femoris, adductors longus, brevis, and magnus)*. Remember, these muscles are typically locked short, overburdened, exhausted, and much neglected. Often, they are the first to report pain signals. The following protocols consist of:

1. Warming the tissue
2. Myofascial release
3. Pin and rock strategy for softening the tissue
4. Direct compression with active movement to clear trigger points

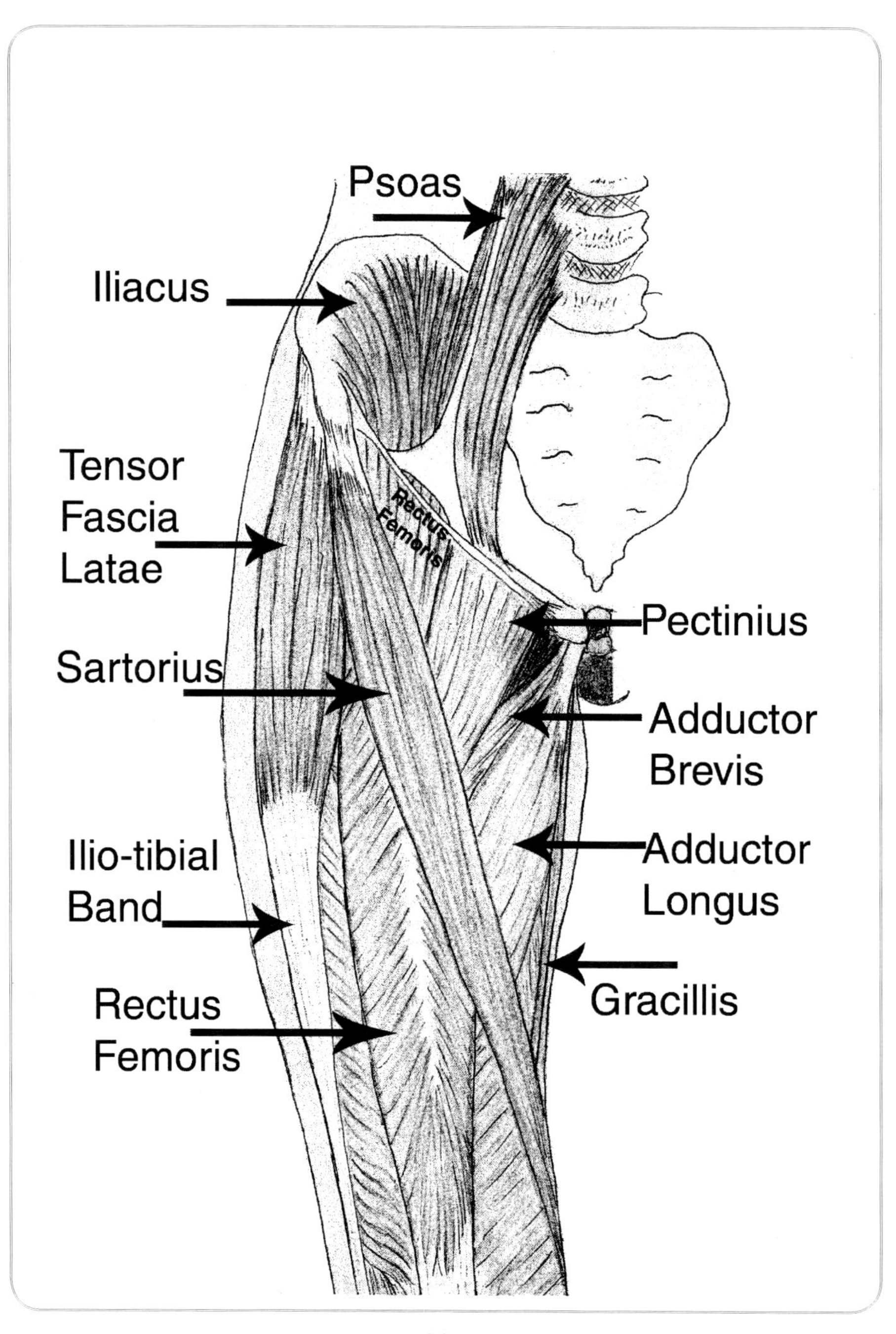

STEP 1:

A. **Warm up** the quads and secondary thigh flexors using a combination of gliding, kneading and compression strokes. Use as little lubricant as possible.

B. **Freeing the fascia:** Our goal is to help restore healthy tissue density and free the fascia of all of the secondary thigh flexors and quadriceps of adhesions and congested areas. Using your finger pads, begin superior and meander your way inferior to aid in freeing the tissue. You'll detour to the right and left, but the general direction will be superior/inferior.

Use a firm yet gentle, sustained pressure, moving slowly through the layers of tissue to assess and release adhesions and thickenings. When you feel a thickened or congested area, or when your fingers stop, unable to drag freely over the tissue, maintain a gentle direct pressure, meeting and melting this barrier, for about 30 seconds to one minute. Ask your client to perform active movement. This movement should be small — we're not looking for a large muscular contraction, just enough to encourage the fascial layers to glide. (See list of possible movements on page 23.) Your fingers will feel a softening of the tissue.

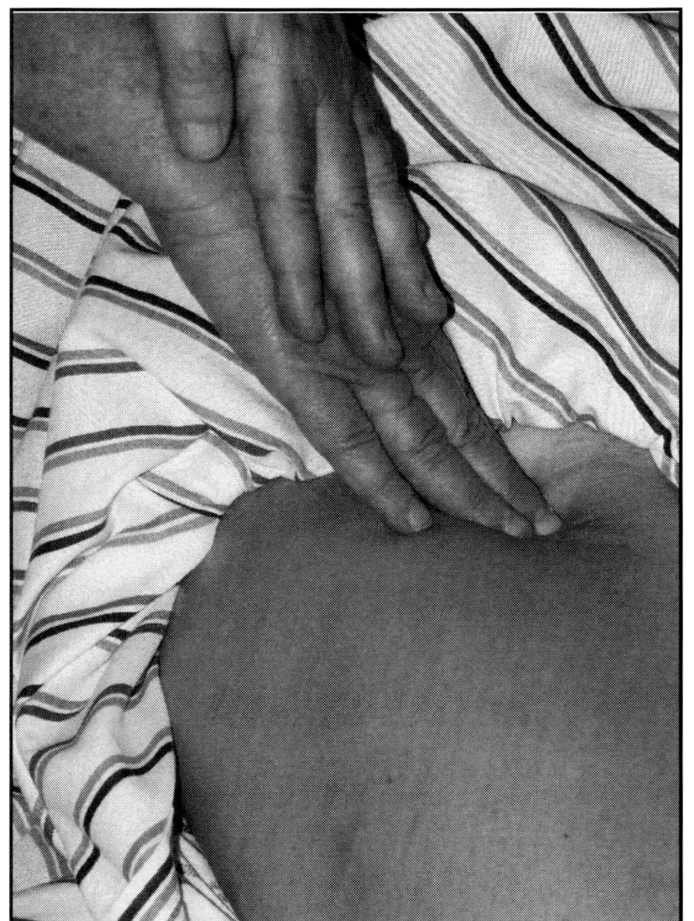

Freeing the fascia – secondary thigh flexors and quadriceps: Use little or no lubricant.

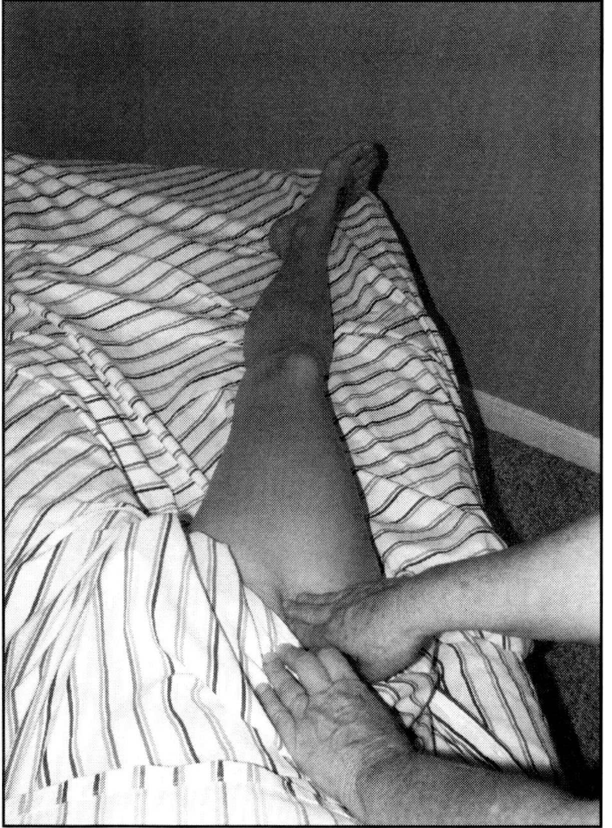

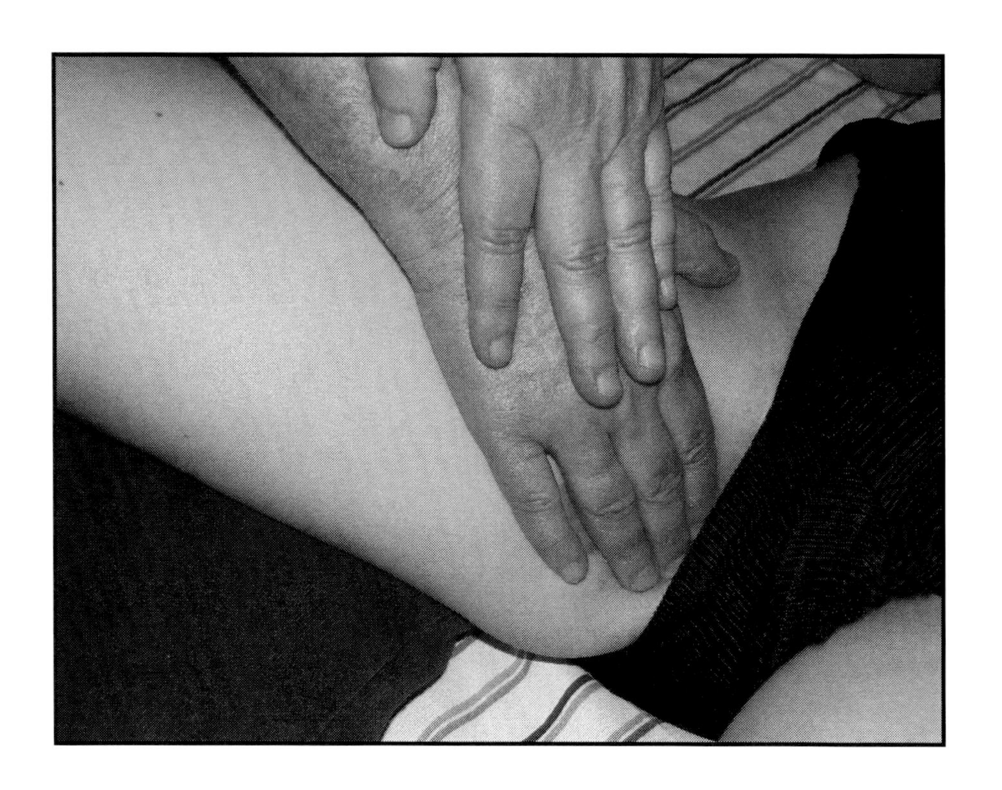

Freeing the fascia: Adductors

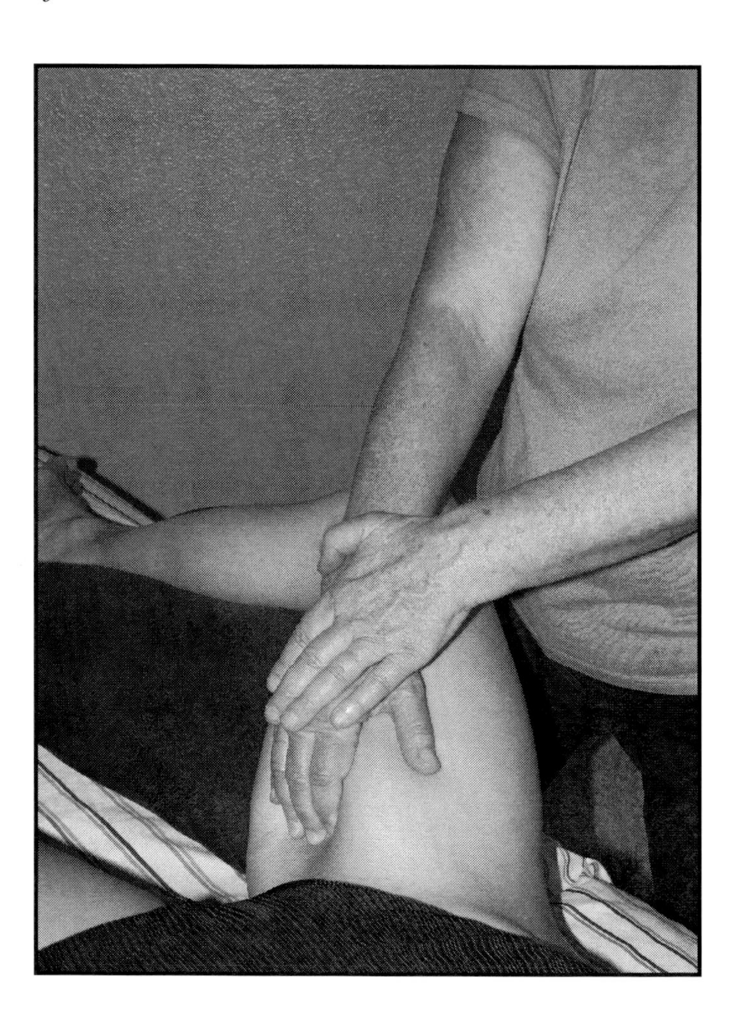

STEP 2:

Trigger point release: Our goal is to clear the *tensor fascia latae, sartorius, pectineus, and rectus femoris* area of obnoxious and pain-producing trigger points. Trigger points are extremely specific; use care to move less than a centimeter between points or you might miss one.

We'll concentrate our work on the area just below the inferior ilium and pubic bones. Start medially and work your way laterally as far as you can go. If this area is really tender, I've found it helpful to place a heat source like a flaxseed pillow or hot stone across the thigh joint before performing deep tissue work. To *decrease* pain/tenderness in this area, slack the muscles by placing a bolster under the knees while working. Avoid pressing on the femoral artery.

Release these secondary thigh flexors with the following strategies:

A. *Pin and Rock*: *Gently* place your elbow, knuckle, small hot stone or other tool into the tissue (you'll be on *pectineus*). **Go to and stop at first barrier — less is more!** Rock the femur back and forth. Rocking is a fabulous portal into muscle tissue because of its immediate relaxation response. Do this *pin and rock* technique all the way across the upper thigh below the inguinal ligament.
Repeat as necessary.

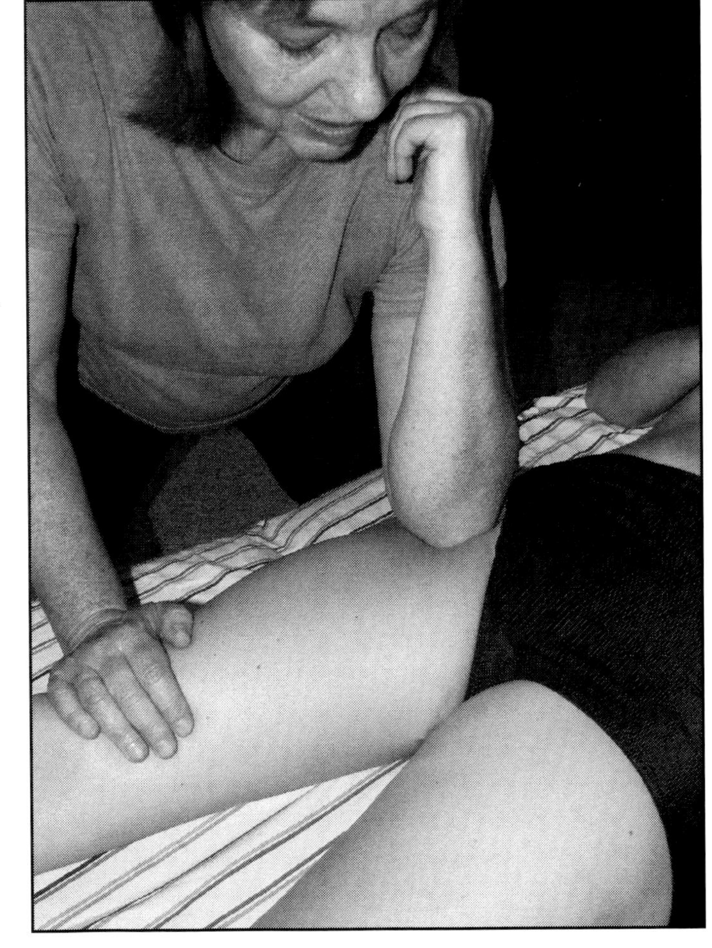

Pin and Rock: Secondary thigh flexors. The therapist's downhill hand (just above the knee) is rocking the femur side to side.

B. ***Muscle Swimming with Active Movement:*** Go back to the medial muscle (*pectineus*) and place your elbow, knuckle, or small tool into the tissue. Ask your client to let you know when you've hit a tender spot/trigger point. Now we'll go muscle swimming, using active movement to penetrate muscle layers and clear trigger points. A list of possible active movements for releasing the secondary thigh flexors includes:

1. Thigh flexions
2. Internal rotation
3. External rotation
4. Abduction
5. Adduction
6. Any combination of the above movements
7. Adding resistance to any of the above movements.
8. Ask your client if she feels any other movement would be helpful

Thigh flexions are a good place to start. Teach your client the movement pattern using passive movement and do it for her several times. Then have her do the movement 4-5 times. Check in with her, asking the question, *"Is there any change?"* Using this language instead of *"Is it better?"* gives your client permission to tell the truth.

If she reports that it is better, you'll know the movement pattern is working. If she reports no change, try adding resistance to the pattern. In the case of thigh flexions, this would involve placing your hand on the front of her thigh during the flexion phase and on the back of her thigh during the extension phase.

If adding resistance does not work, try another movement pattern. This is where this work gets interesting; the trial and error of experimenting with different movements and levels of resistance develops our skills and intuition.

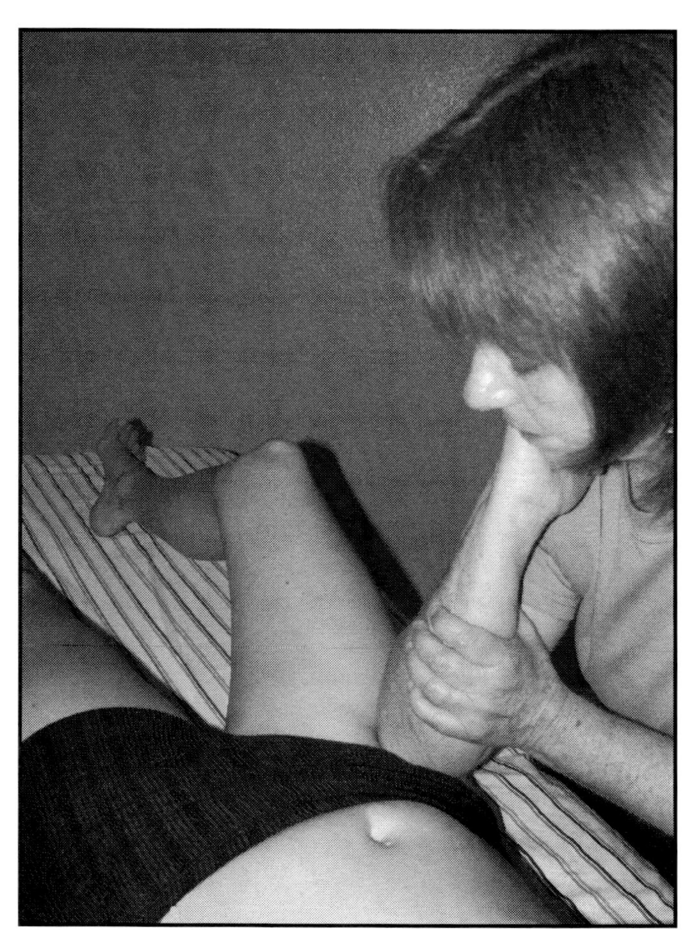

Above: Pinning a trigger point while the client does active thigh flexions.

Reminder: Whenever you sense tension and guarding in your client, decrease your pressure and add gentle rocking.

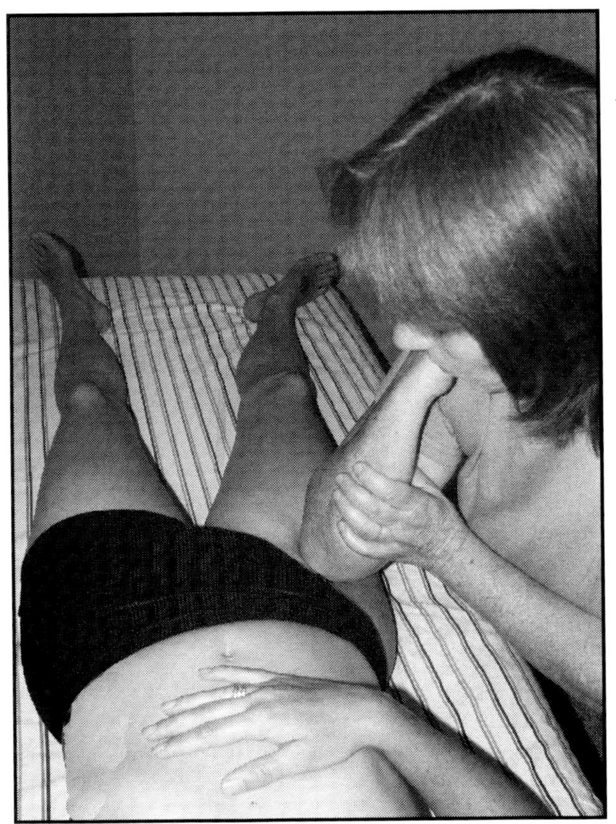

Left: Pinning a trigger point while the client does active external rotation (right leg)

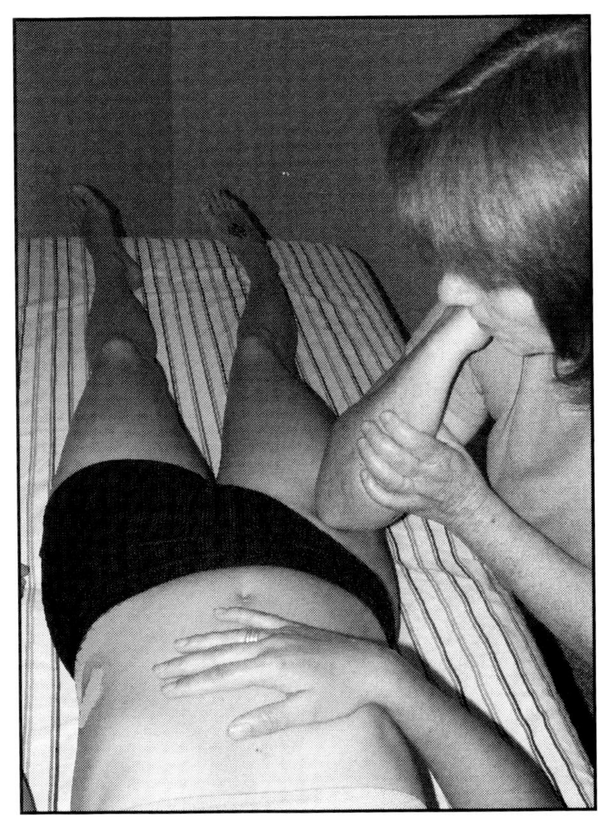

Right: Pinning a trigger point while the client does active internal rotation (right leg)

Protocols for Releasing the Iliopsoas

Now we dive into the mysterious and complex iliopsoas. Keep in mind that slow is better and less is more. The following protocols consist of:

1. Warming the abdominal muscles
2. Iliopsoas location test
3. Warming the iliopsoas with the Pin and Rock strategy to soften the tissue
4. Direct compression with active movement to clear trigger points

STEP 1:
Have client bend her knees to slacken the muscles. Release the abdominal muscles using gentle compressions and kneading strokes. We need to go *deep* to the abdominal muscles to access the iliopsoas. People often carry quite a bit of tension in the abdominals; you may find that this softening of the abdominals may take some time. Working through a sheet for both the abdominals and the iliopsoas takes some of the "charge" out of the work for the client. Working through the sheet is fine — it's impossible to get the nails short enough!

STEP 2:
A. Place fingers of one or two hands at lowest part of iliac crest, just medial to the bone. Slide under the abdominals. You'll be in the bowl or concave area called the external iliac fossa on the *iliacus* muscle, just medial and superior to where you released the secondary thigh flexors. Follow the contour of the iliac fossa — it will guide you to the deeper tissue. **Muscle test to confirm you are on the *iliacus*** Ask your client to flex the thigh while you apply resistance with your hand or elbow. You should feel the muscle "pop out" into your hand.

B. Now slide your fingers medially to palpate the ***psoas.*** It feels like a long, wide sausage. Repeat the resisted thigh flexion to check your location.

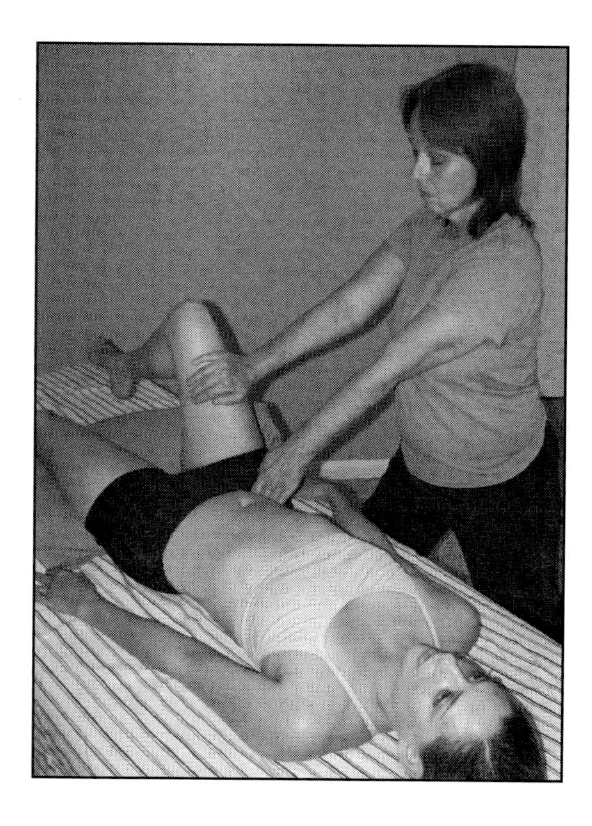

Checking the location of the iliopsoas with resisted thigh flexions.

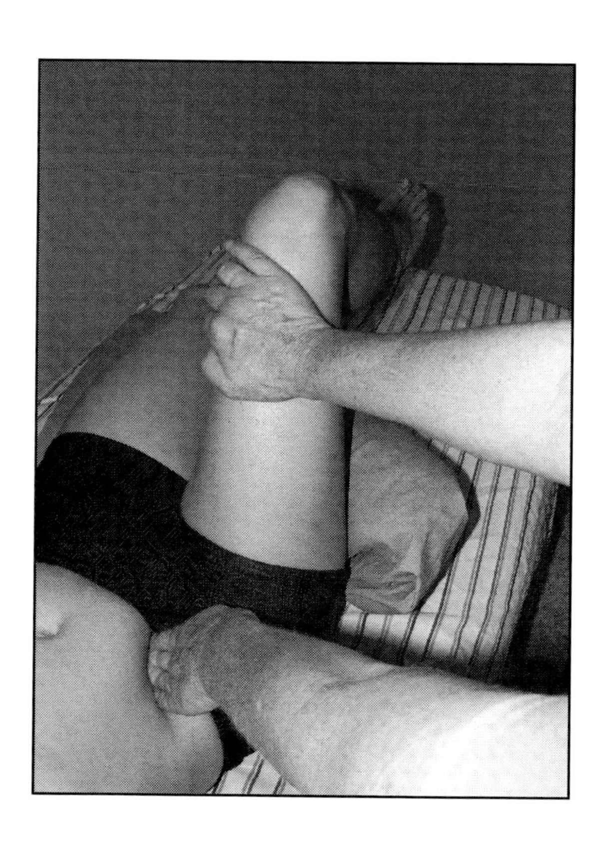

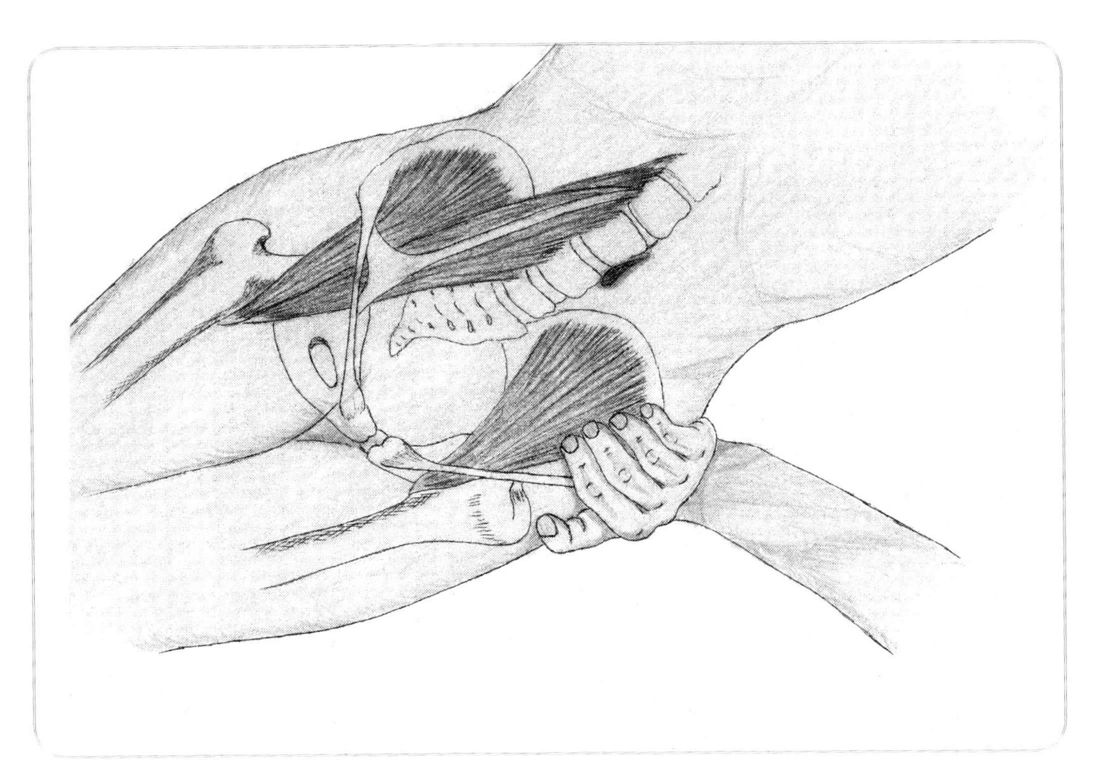

Above: the right side of the graphic shows the therapist's fingers on the iliacus. The left side shows both psoas and iliacus. You can see that to palpate the psoas, your fingers must slide towards the spine. The psoas has been removed on the right side of the graphic for visibility.

STEP 3:
Pin and Rock

Once you have verified your location, slowly press down into the tissue using a gentle, circular motion, sensing rather than doing. Place your downhill hand on your client's knees and move them side to side, like windshield wipers. This rocking movement relaxes both the tissue and the client as you warm the tissue. Warm up the medial and lateral sections up to the iliac crest with this pin and rock strategy.

Feel for knots, adhesions, and trigger points as you warm the tissue. No need to release them yet. We'll get to that later. Right now, you are assessing the tissue with a **gentle** pressure and getting the client used to your presence in this vulnerable area.

STEP 4:

Muscle Swimming with Active Movement

Once the tissue is warm and receptive, go back to the inferior portion of iliopsoas. Now we'll work to release knots, adhesions, and trigger points with our Muscle Swimming with Active Movement. When you feel a knot, adhesion, or trigger point, gently pin the area while the client does active movement.

A list of possible active movements for releasing the iliopsoas includes:

1. "Windshield wipers" (the client sways her knees from side to side with feet planted on the table and knees bent)
2. Spinal rotation: instruct your client to let her knees fall all the way to the left as you work the iliopsoas from this position of spinal rotation. Repeat with spinal rotation to the right.
3. Thigh flexions
4. Pelvic tilts
5. Deep breathing with the emphasis on a longer exhale than usual.
6. Ask your client if she feels any other movement would be helpful
7. Any combination of the above movements
8. Adding resistance to any of the above movements. This loads the muscle and recruits more fibers, allowing you to swim through the myofascial tissue.

Work the medial and lateral portions of the muscle. Hooking your fingers under the crest is effective for the lateral portion (iliacus). Combine static compression, rocking, and myofascial release to the length and width of the muscle. Slowly work your way superiorly. We work inferior to superior because the inferior section is easiest to access.

Reminder: Give your client a break! Working on these muscles, especially the iliopsoas, can be quite stressful. Incorporate what I call the "sweet stuff" during your deep tissue work, i.e., energy work, a short foot massage, some relaxing effleurage, etc.

Below: releasing the iliopsoas while the client does "windshield wipers"

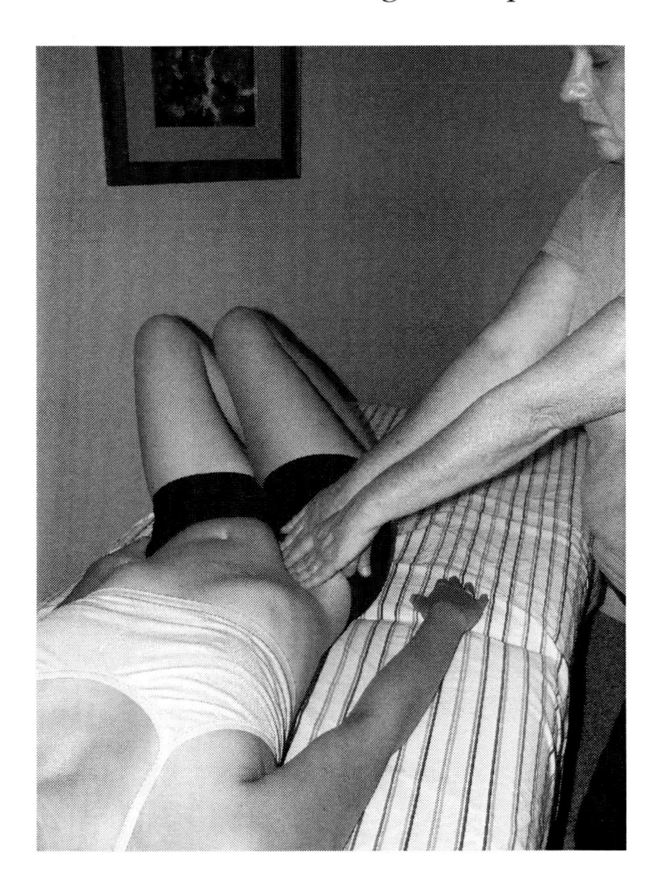

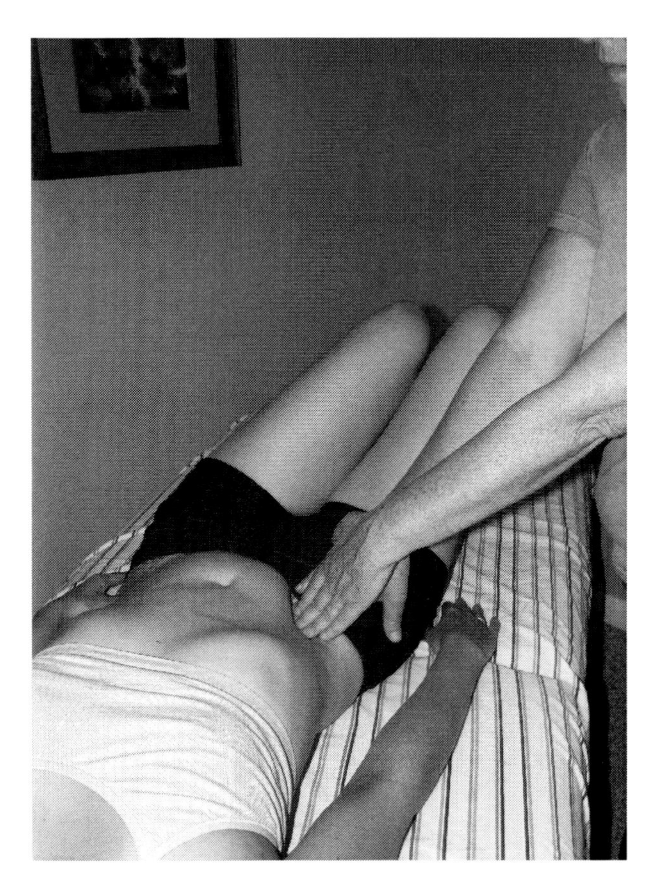

"Windshield wipers"* are a good place to start because the swaying movement is easy and relaxing and you've just done it during the warm-up. Have your client do the movement 4-5 times. Check in with her, asking the question, *"Is there any change?"* Using this language instead of *"Is it better?"* gives your client permission to tell the truth. If she reports that it is better, you'll know the movement pattern is working. If she reports no change, try adding resistance to the pattern. If adding resistance still yields no results, try another movement pattern from the list. Teach your client the movement pattern using passive movement and do it for her several times, then go to an active movement pattern.

*"Windshield wipers" can easily become spinal rotation just by letting the legs fall completely to one side.

On the following pages you'll find photos of different movement patterns.

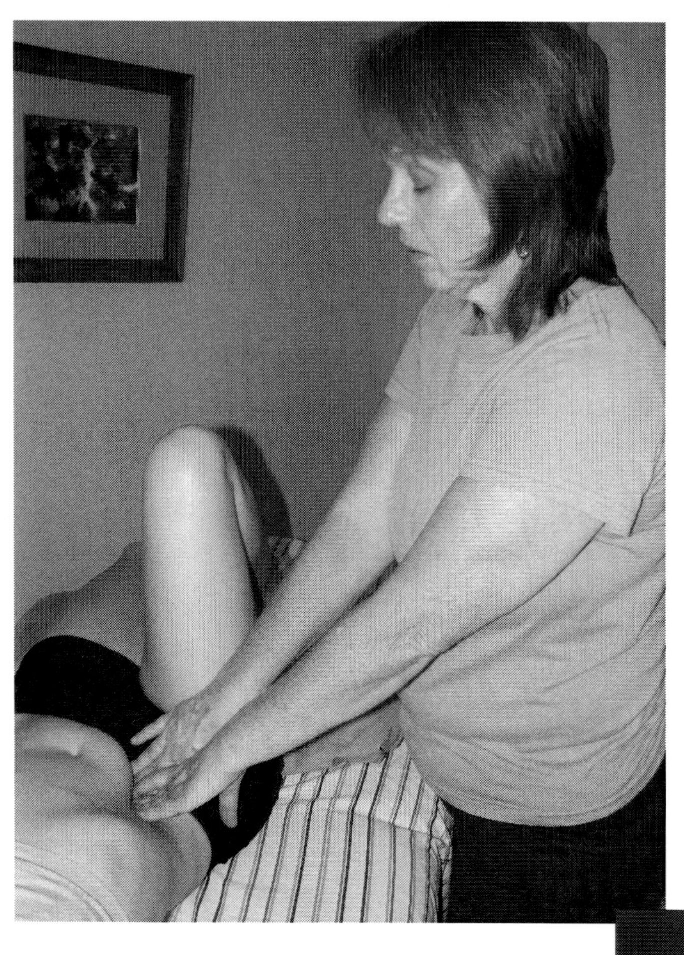

Left: pinning the iliopsoas as the client does active thigh flexions.

Pinning the iliopsoas as the client does active pelvic tilts.

Photo right: Client doing anterior pelvic tilt.

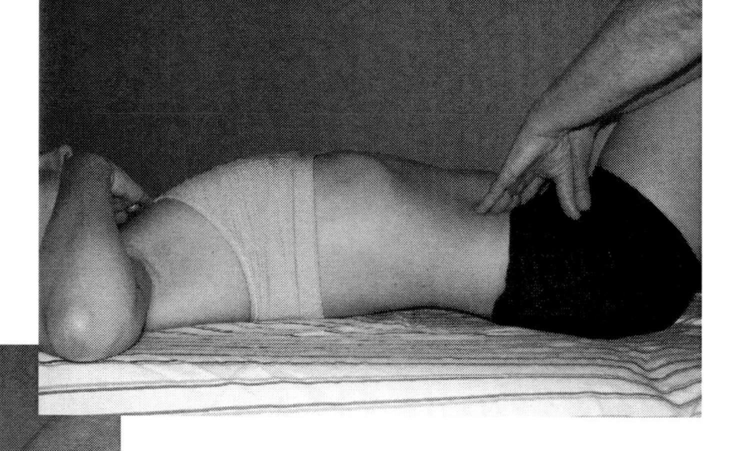

Photo left: Client doing posterior pelvic tilt.

STEP 5:
When you arrive at the ASIS, you'll be entering the *superior psoas* territory and you'll need to change your entry to go more medially toward the spine.

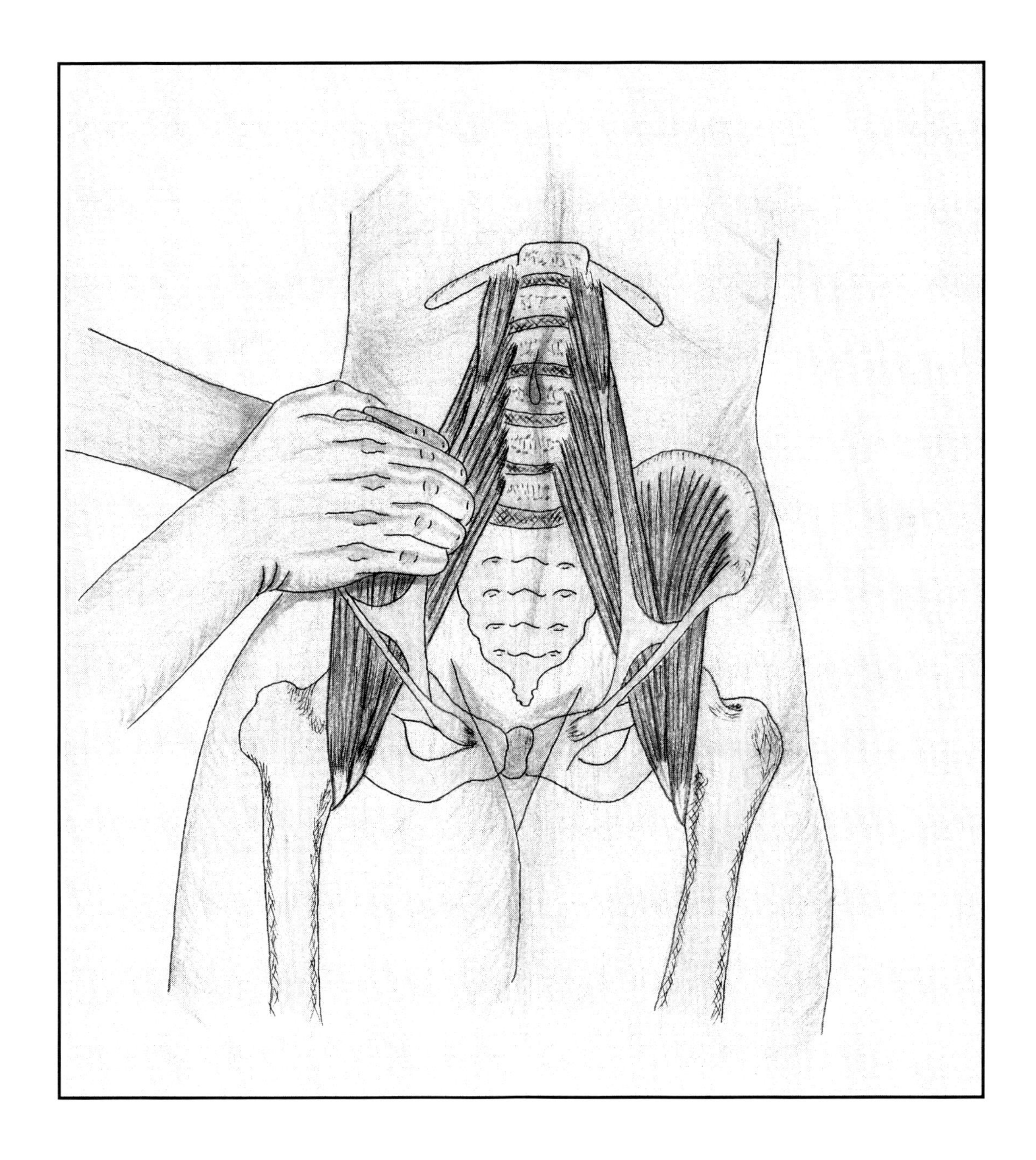

Reminder: Movement (active and passive) allows you to work through the muscle layers.

A. Place the client's leg in external rotation and abduction and rest it on a pillow. This position facilitates palpation of the medial portion of this superior section of the psoas. Press the fingers of one hand down and medially under the abdominal muscles. To verify you are on the *psoas*, have the client flex the femur. If you feel the muscle contracting, bingo, you're on it! It should feel like a large sausage. *Be extra gentle and cautious on this superior section —be vigilant that you are on muscle tissue and not neurovascular structures. Go slow and listen to the tissue.*

B. Because the fibers of the psoas interweave with the fascia of the diaphragm, the deep breathing technique with the emphasis on a longer exhale than usual can be quite effective here. Slowly work your way superiorly up as high as T12. It's easy to "lose" the muscle the higher you go. With practice you'll be able to stay on it. Work as high as you can to release the fascial adhesions that often form in this vulnerable area. Most therapists only work the lower part of the psoas, omitting this crucial area.

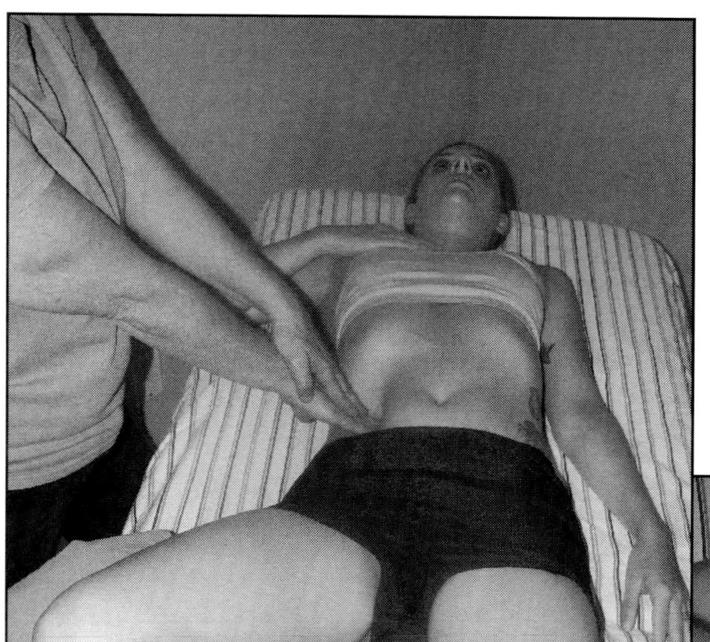

Releasing the superior portion of the psoas

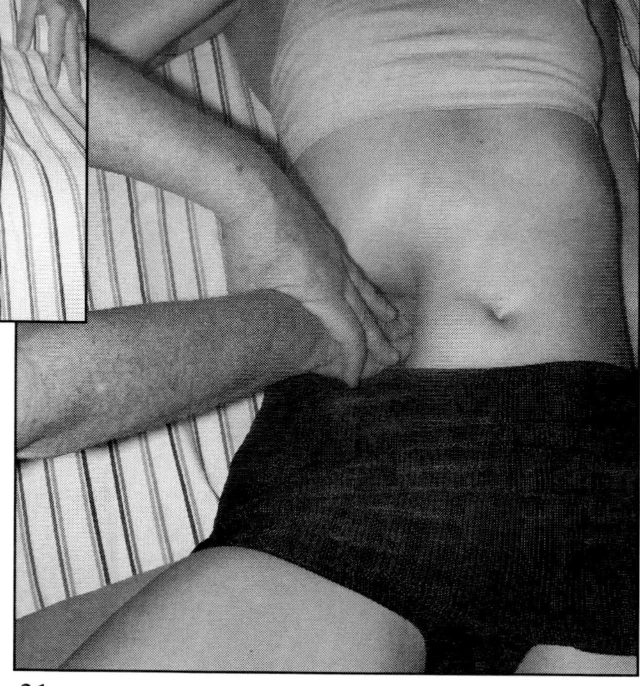

STEP 6:
The photo below shows the therapist gently touching the iliopsoas and quadratus lumborum at the same time. Think of this step as an energetic reminder to the muscles that they work together. Sometimes a profound release happens in this step. If the tissue is open enough, you can work deeper. As always, *be gentle, go slow and listen to the tissue.*

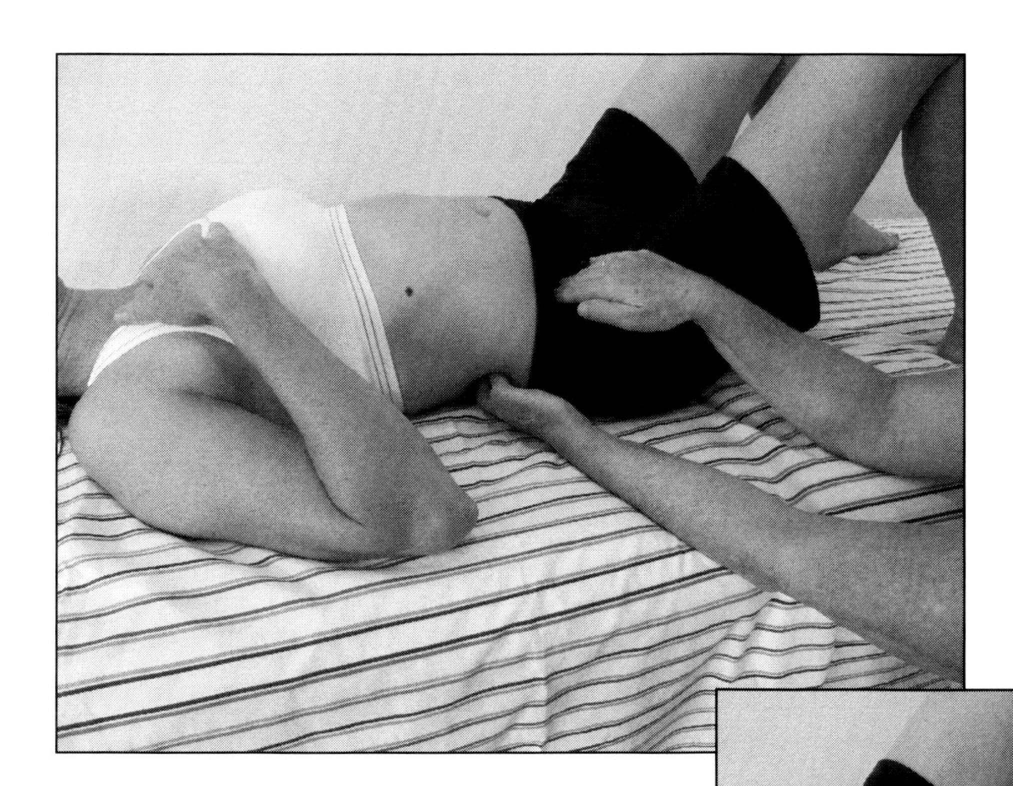

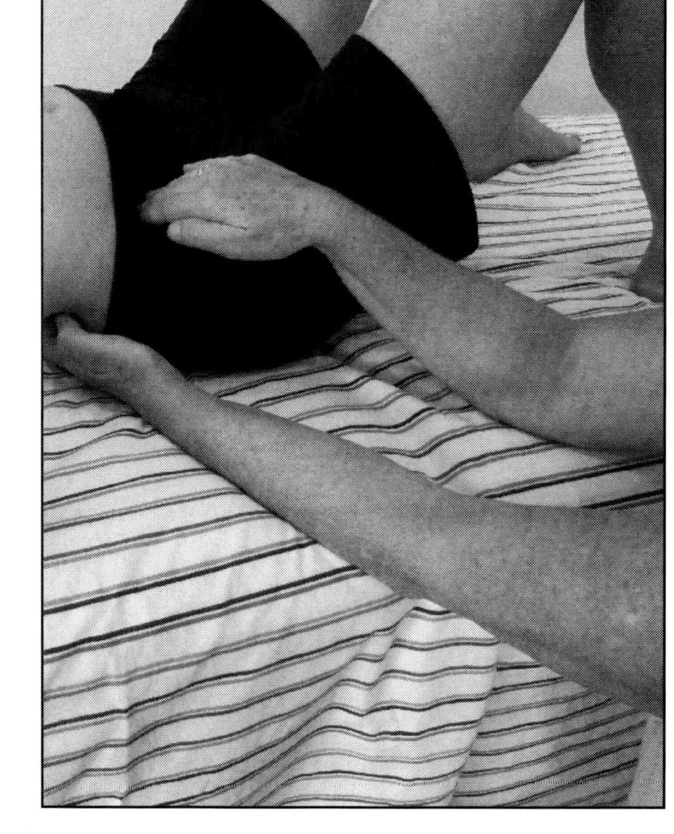

Releasing the iliopsoas and quadratus lumborum at the same time

STEP 7: Iliopsoas/thigh flexor stretches

These muscles can be stretched from supine, side-lying, and prone. Stretch the muscle after you work it. This is when the muscle is most responsive.
The prone version is not included because of the compression on the lumbar discs it causes in many people. I always have my clients get dressed for the supine version of this stretch since it's impossible to do with a drape!

Take the muscle(s) slightly beyond the natural end point of the range of motion into the "stretch zone". This end point is called the physiological barrier. Hold the stretch for a minimum of 15 seconds (3-4 deep breaths), encouraging the client to "breathe into" the stretch. After you have held the stretch for 15 seconds, see if the muscle will comfortably respond to an additional stretch. You can do two or three repetitions of the stretch as needed. Maximum benefit is reached at about 90 seconds. Again, encourage your client to tell you if you're going too far or not far enough.

If your client's tissue is fighting the stretch, it's usually because the resting length is so short and the stretch reflex is being engaged. PNF (Proprioceptive Neuromuscular Facilitation) strategies such as antagonist and agonist contract are great tactics for reducing the signaling of the stretch reflex. You can also try using a 2-3 second stretch with more repetitions.

Ask your client to give you verbal feedback about the stretching. This is crucial to avoid activating the stretch reflex. First ask her where is she feeling the stretch. The stretch should be felt in the muscle that's being stretched or in what I call the "neighborhood association". In stretching the iliopsoas, your client could feel that stretch in any of the nine thigh flexors or even in the abdominal muscles. **She should not feel it in the low back.** That's a red flag that something is wrong, usually a stabilization issue that can be resolved with a prop.

Clients who are swaybacked or feel back pain in this position generally need a pillow under the neck for support. **Pelvic stabilization is a key issue in this stretch.** Keep a keen eye out for anterior tilting of the pelvis. You can provide stabilization with your hand or give your client movement cues so she can provide stabilization. I like to coach my clients to find those deep pelvic/abdominal stabilizers before intervening and providing stabilization. Here's a couple of movement cues to suggest to your clients:

1. Ask her to gently press her low back towards the table.
2. Ask her to imagine that a heavy pillow is resting on her belly. This engages the pelvic stabilizers.
3. Place a flax seed pillow or something like it that has some weight on your client's belly.

On the following pages you'll find a number of variations of the supine version of the stretch as well as a side-lying iliopsoas/thigh flexor stretch.

SUPINE ILIOPSOAS/THIGH FLEXOR STRETCH

Step 1: Gently traction the femur, then press the leg to be stretched towards the floor into hyperextension. This also stretches the secondary thigh flexors: ***rectus femoris*, *tensor fascia latae, sartorius, pectineus, gracilis, adductors longus, brevis, and magnus***.

Step 2: Hold for 15-30 seconds. To use a PNF strategy, have the client push up to engage/shorten the thigh flexors with no more than 20% effort. Client holds the contraction for 8-10 seconds. Therapist then feels if the tissue can stretch farther. Repeat the PNF two more times. PNF techniques are especially good for re-educating the stretch reflex and reducing its signaling on tissue that has an especially short resting length.

Step 3: Experiment with rotating the femur internally and externally to stretch different fibers of these muscles (shown on next two pages).

Step 4: To come out of the stretch, lift the leg back onto the table, so the client does not engage the muscle.

For those clients who can't hold their own leg, a variation is for the client to put the opposite foot on the therapist's shoulder (see photo below.)

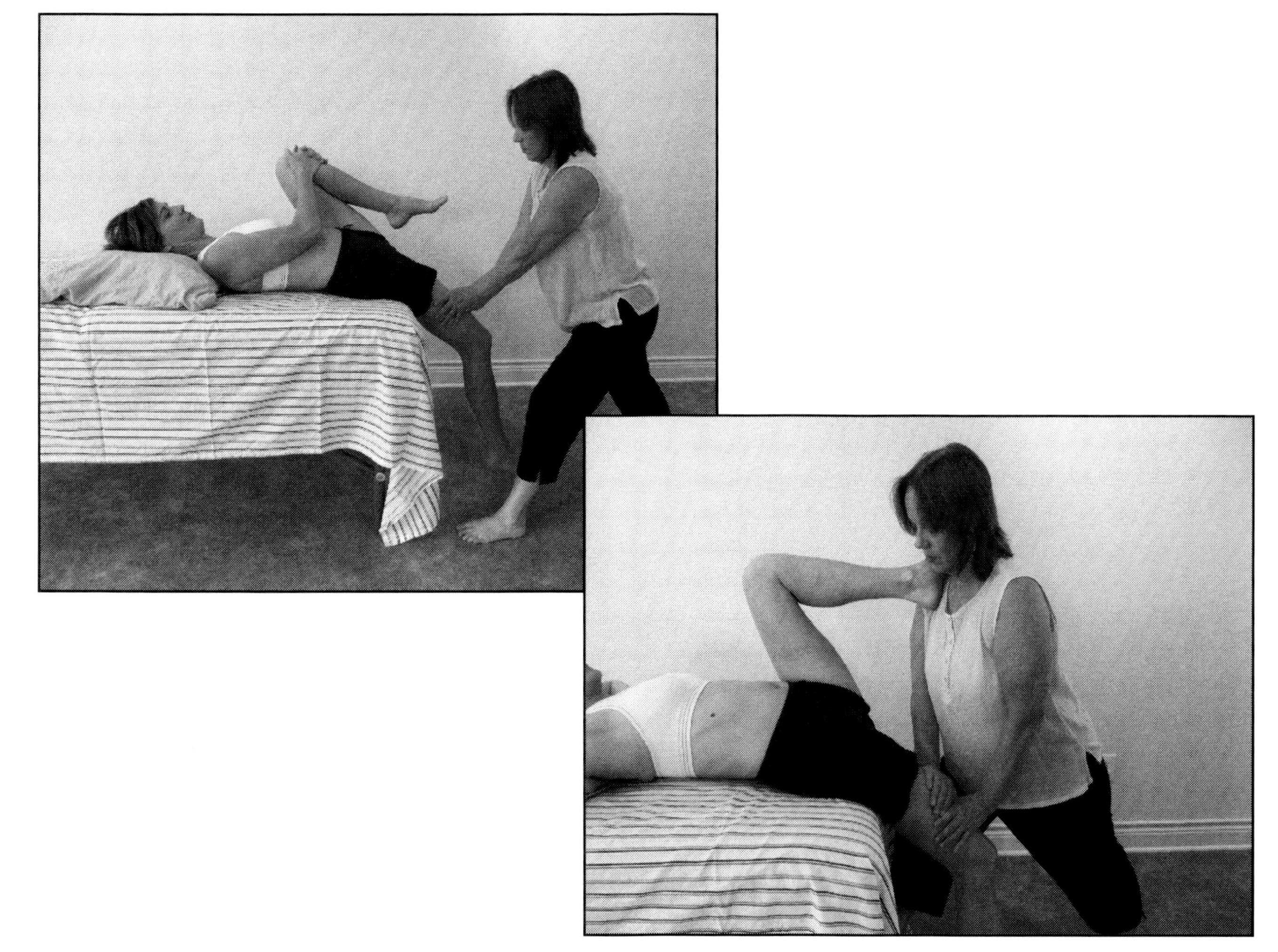

SUPINE ILIOPSOAS/THIGH FLEXOR STRETCH VARIATIONS

For those clients who cannot self-stabilize their pelvis, the therapist can stabilize it for them by placing a hand on the same side pelvis and exerting a gentle pressure toward the table. You can do this stabilizing maneuver with any of the variations.

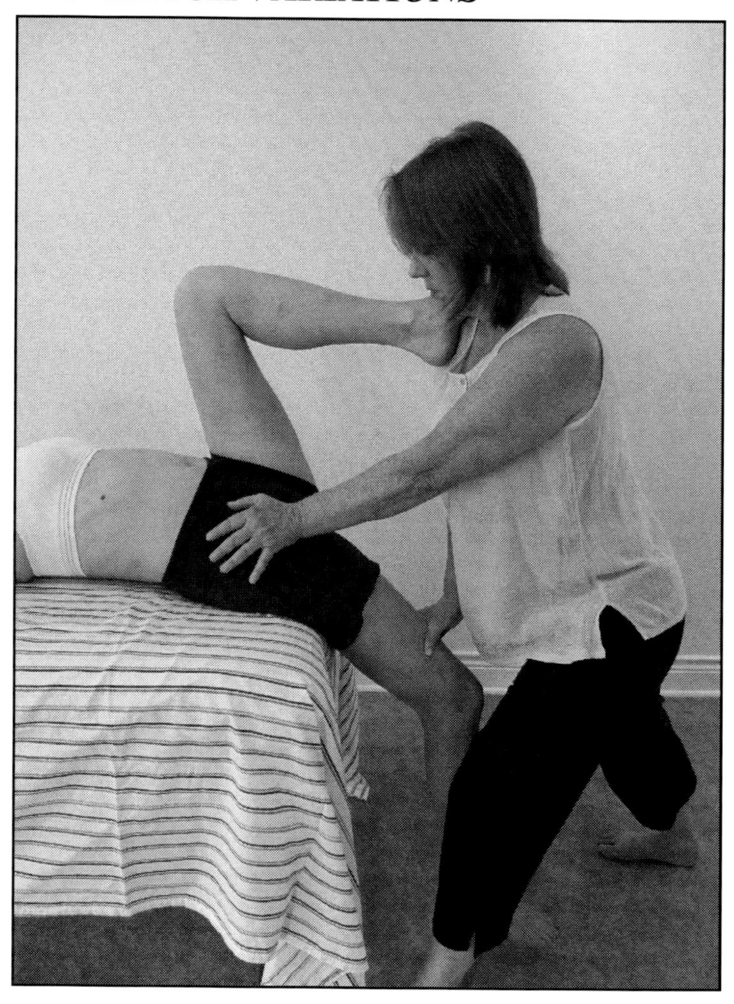

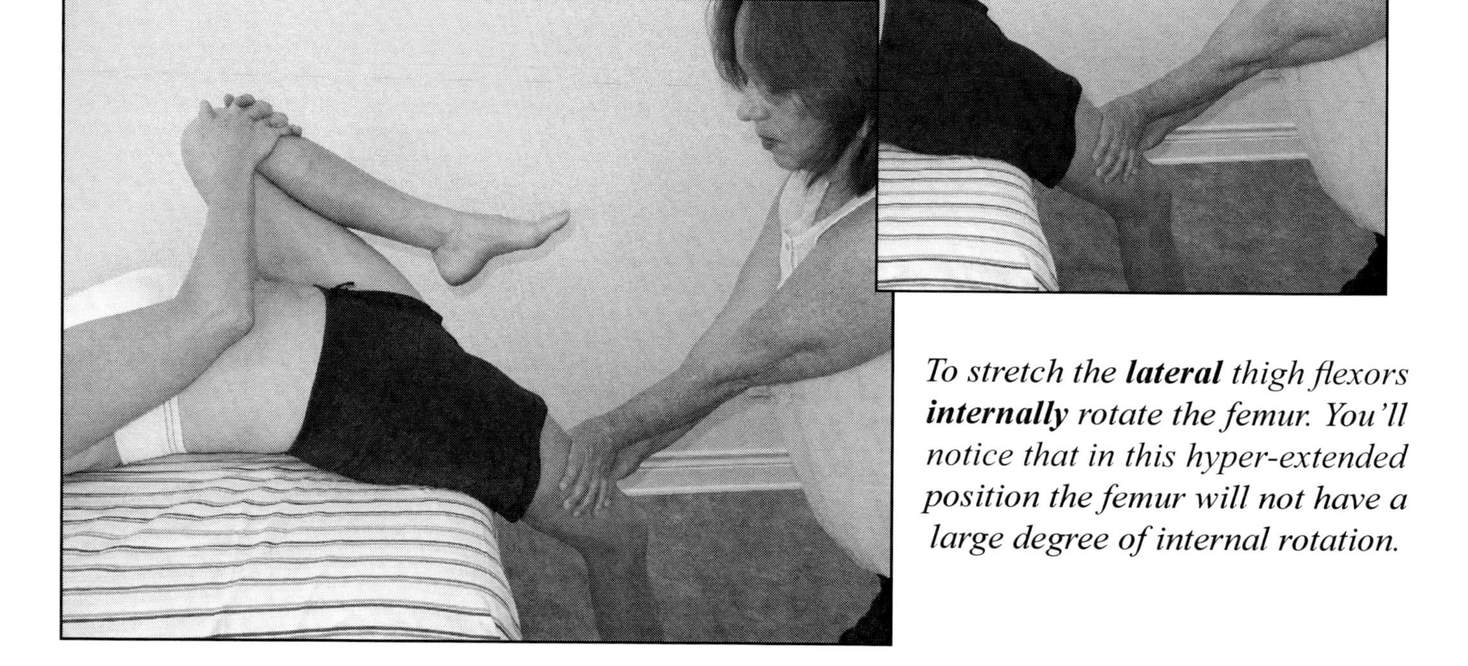

*To stretch the **lateral** thigh flexors **internally** rotate the femur. You'll notice that in this hyper-extended position the femur will not have a large degree of internal rotation.*

SUPINE ILIOPSOAS/THIGH FLEXOR STRETCH VARIATIONS

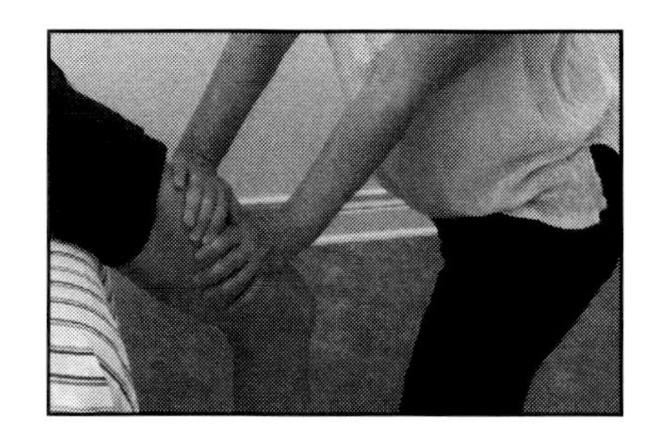

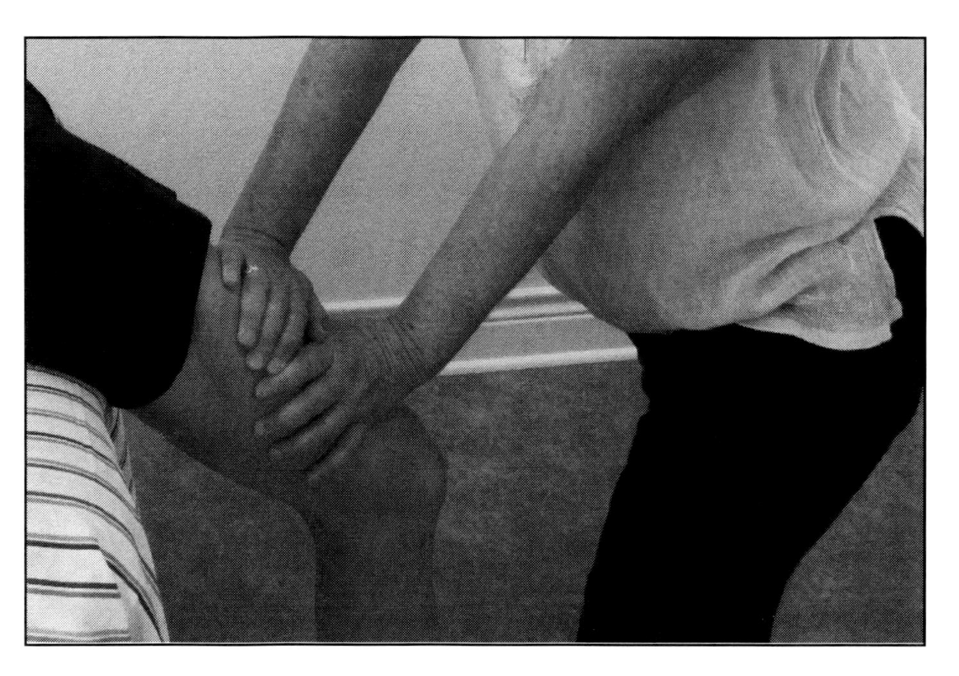

*Above: To stretch the **medial** thigh flexors, **externally** rotate the femur. You'll notice that in this hyper-extended position the femur will not have a large degree of external rotation.*

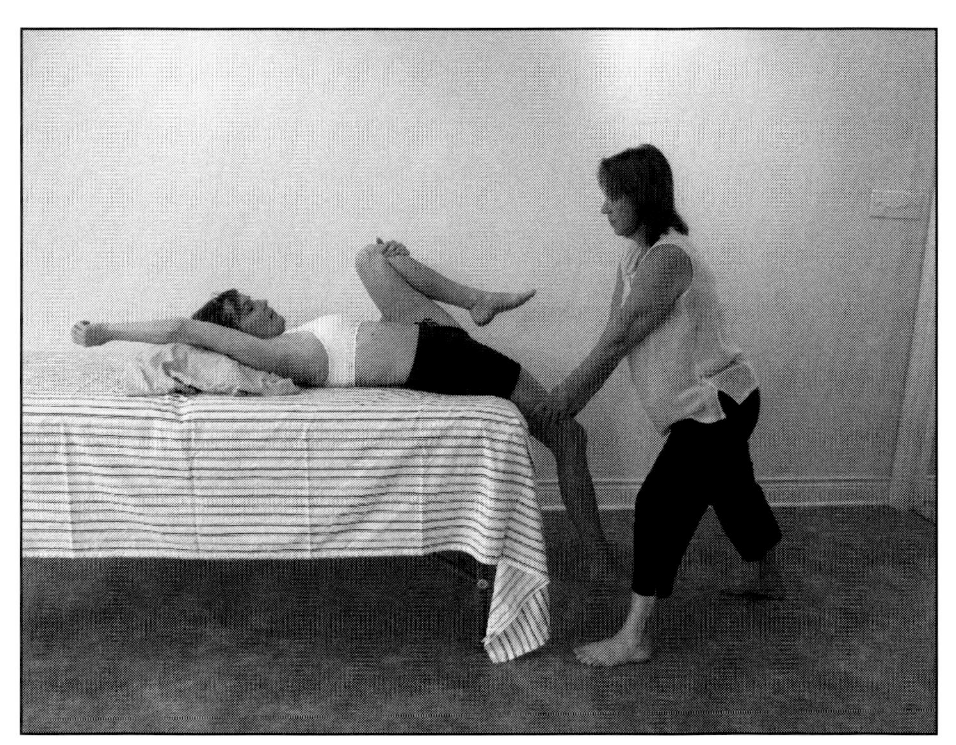

To include the abdominals and latissimus dorsi in this stretch, ask your client to reach the same side arm over her head.

SUPINE ILIOPSOAS/THIGH FLEXOR STRETCH VARIATIONS

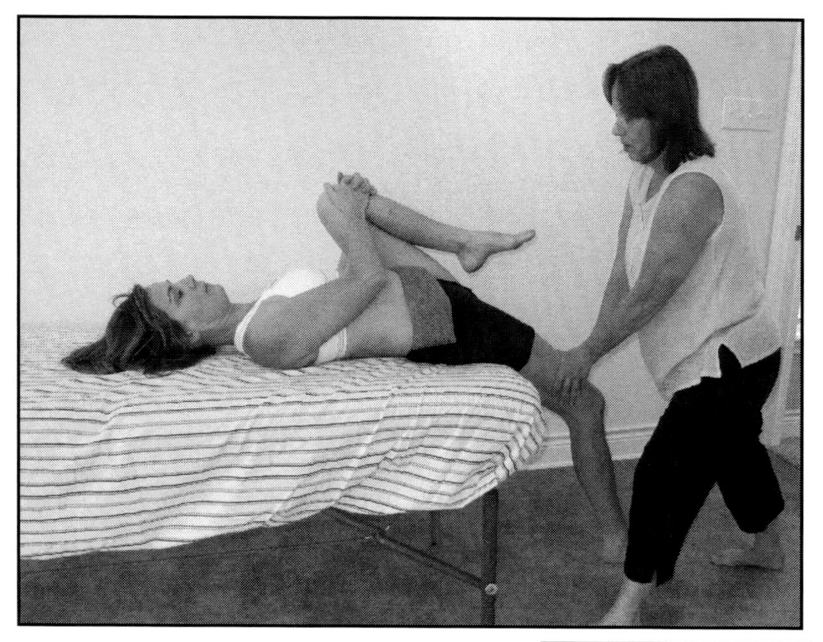

Left: Using a flax seed pillow to encourage pelvic stabilization.

Right: You can do additional release work on the iliopsoas during the stretch. Be gentle! Working a muscle in a stretched state usually is the most painful state to work it in. However, your client may need to have the muscle worked in a stretched state to get a complete release.

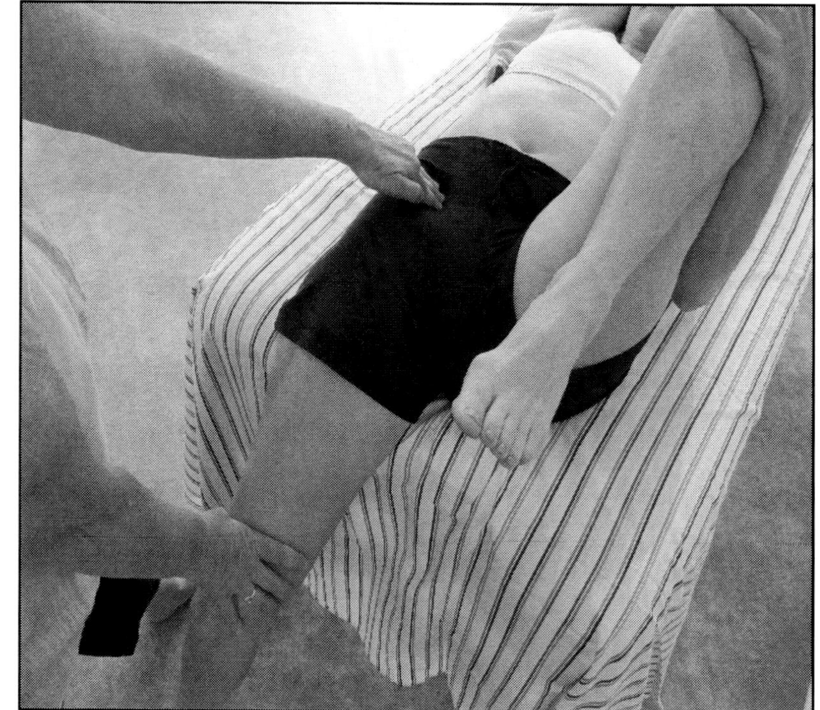

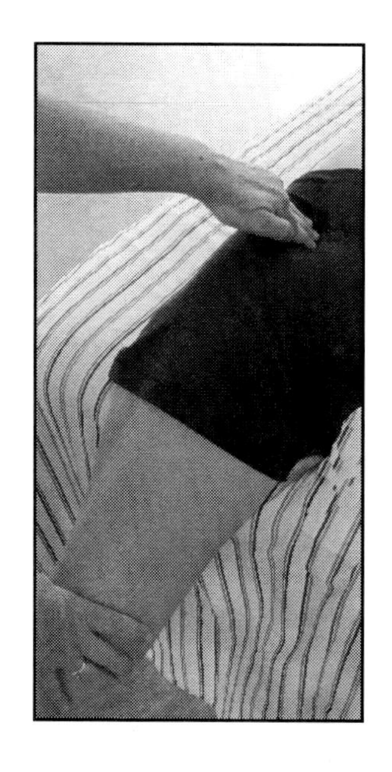

SIDE-LYING ILIOPSOAS/THIGH FLEXOR STRETCH

The technique for a side-lying iliopsoas/thigh flexor stretch is the same as the protocol for the posterior pelvic tilt correction but with a different emphasis. In the correction, the emphasis is on a repositioning of bones. Here our emphasis will be on lengthening the muscles and surrounding fascia.

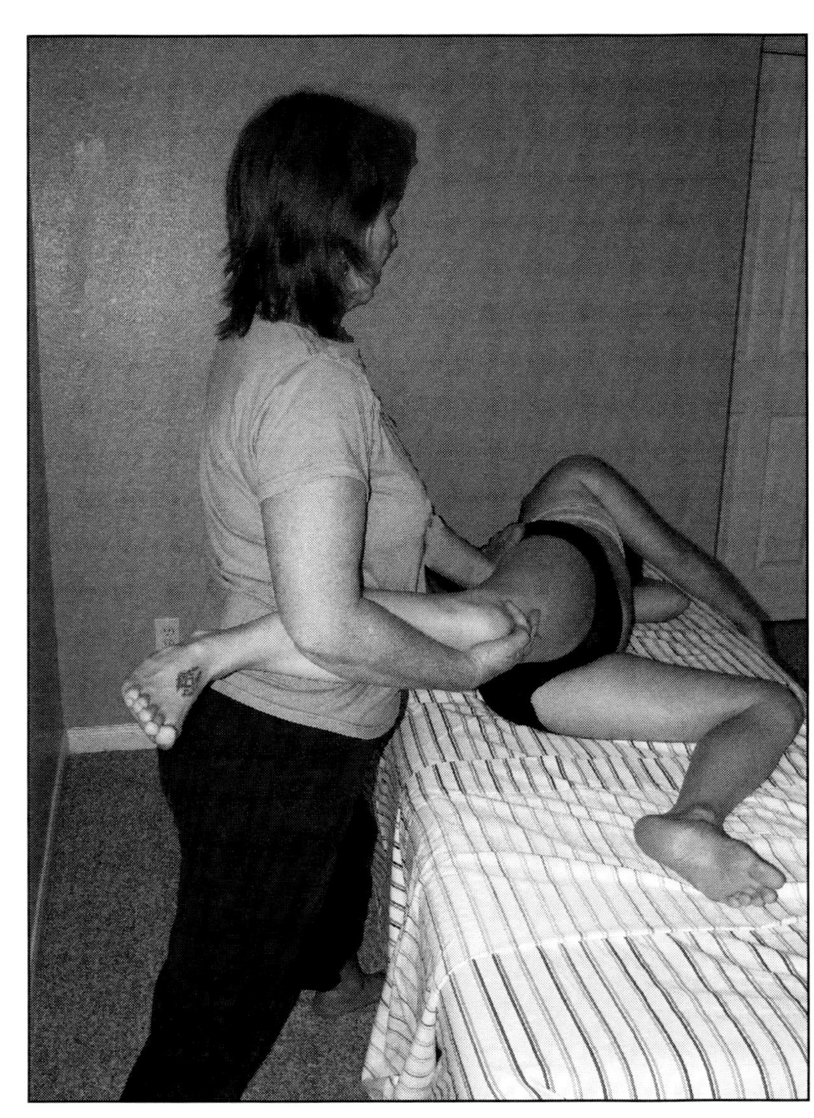

Step 1: Ask your client to bend her knee and flex the thigh of the bottom leg to stabilize the pelvis.

Step 2: Hyperextend the top leg as far back as comfortably possible to provide a gentle lengthening of the iliopsoas/thigh flexors. You may wrap the leg around your waist to help hold the weight of the leg. Your uphill hand should be pushing up on the ischium as your other hand pulls the top leg back into hyperextension.

Step 3: PNF - if needed for a very short resting length: Ask your client to gently flex the thigh isometrically as you provide resistance. Have them hold the contraction for 6-8 seconds, then relax.

Step 4: Increase the hyperextension. Hold for 15 seconds and repeat.

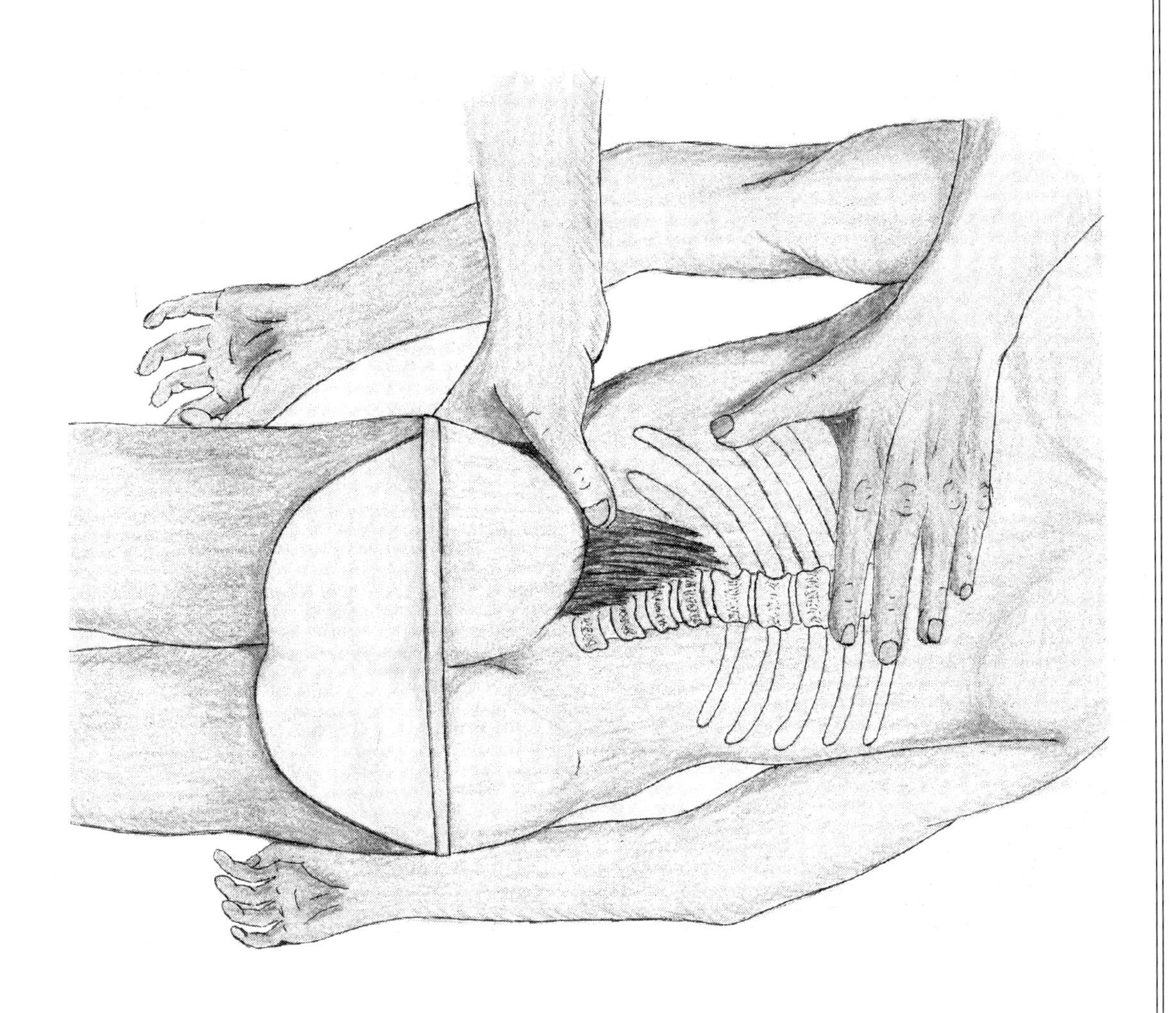

QUADRATUS LUMBORUM

Attachments: (above) 12th rib and lumbar vertebrae 1-4; (below) ilium and iliolumbar ligament.
Actions: lateral flexion of the spine; elevation of the ipsilateral ilium (hip hiking); contributes to extension of the spine; stabilizes the 12th rib during inhalation and forced exhalation; plays a significant role in maintaining upright posture.

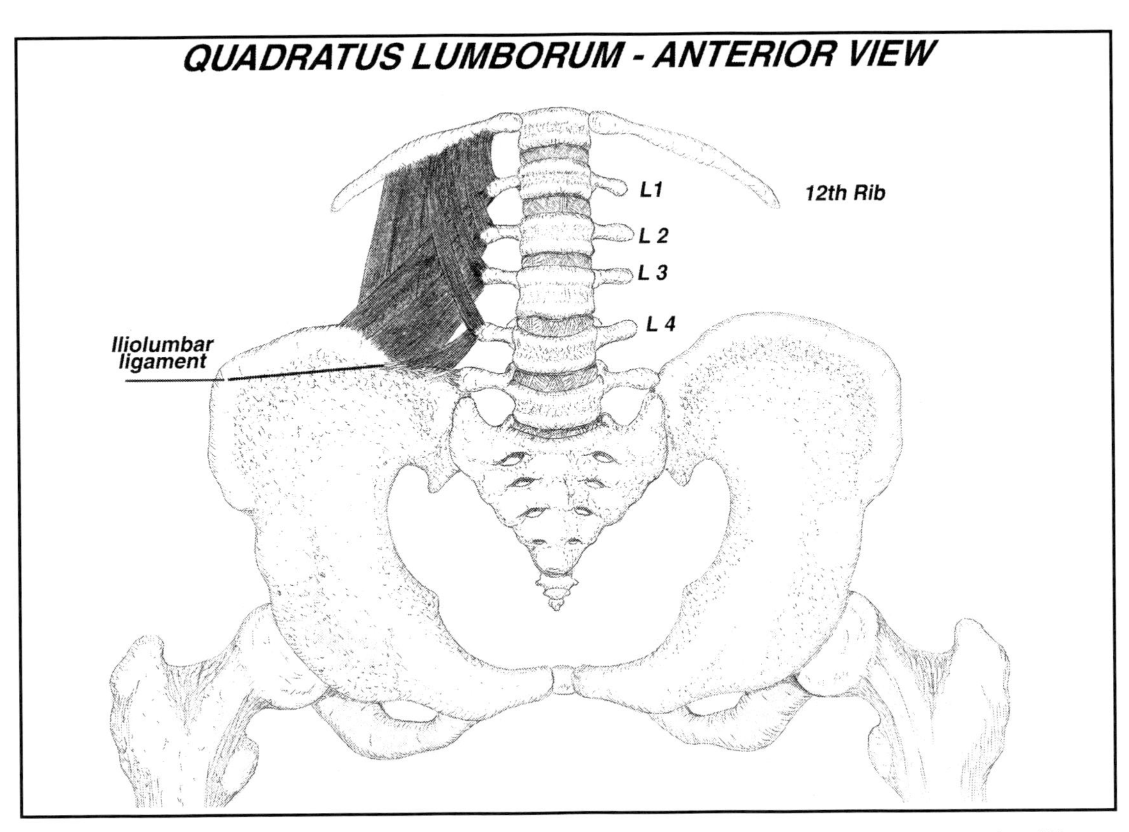

The short, thick quadratus lumborum (QL) is a wonder of a muscle. While the iliopsoas initiates walking, the quadratus lumborum provides the powerful stability so we *can* walk. Some researchers believe that complete bilateral paralysis of the quadratus lumborum would make walking impossible, even with braces. This magnificent muscle is an essential component in the bedrock of our bipedal freedom.

The two QLs work as a team, along with the iliopsoas and lumbar paraspinals (multifidi, erector spinae) in stabilizing the lumbar spine. Like the iliopsoas, if this fundamental stabilizer is distressed it can be like a hurricane blowing through with devastating effects. Any movement can be painful, including urination and defecation. The pain may be excruciating in any position that increases weight bearing and requires stabilization of the lumbar spine. Rolling onto either side from a supine position is painful and difficult; coughing and sneezing can be agonizing. In fact, bending forward, twisting, and sneezing or coughing at the same time can throw the quadratus lumborum into spasm. If it's not a full-blown hurricane, an irritated quadratus lumborum can blow an ill wind of persistent aching pain and gradual loss of lower back and pelvic flexibility, range of motion, and vitality.

Nature has assigned the heavy burden of stabilization to our friend, the dependable quadratus lumborum. She has given it the power and might to do this job by designing an intricate and interlacing fiber arrangement. The most lateral fibers, which are the easiest to palpate, are the nearly vertical iliocostal fibers. The iliolumbar fibers span diagonally from the ilium and iliolumbar ligament to the transverse processes of L1- L4. The diagonal lumbarcostal fibers attach to the 12th rib and the lumbar transverse processes. Keep this complex fiber arrangement in mind as you lovingly work the quadratus lumborum.

Trigger points are often found in both QLs and refer in a horizontal pattern across the lumbar spine, as opposed to the vertical, ipsilateral pattern of the iliopsoas. Trigger points also refer the SI joint, upper sacral region, greater trochanter and lateral thigh, groin, obliques, and buttocks. An improperly functioning quadratus lumborum will affect all the hip/lower back muscles, and secondary trigger points may develop in the gluteus medius and minimus, piriformis, and iliopsoas. Activation of trigger points/dysfunction of the quadratus lumborum can be brought on by numerous factors – a short list includes pregnancy, car accident, weak and/or incorrectly trained abdominal muscles *(see section on client education for suggestions on how to properly train the abdominals)* and short upper arms (elbows that do not reach the iliac crest and cannot reach most armrests. The client tends to lean to one side, placing an eccentric load on the opposite quadratus lumborum. I've noticed that most people's elbows do not reach their iliac crests, so who are the chair manufacturers making chairs for?)

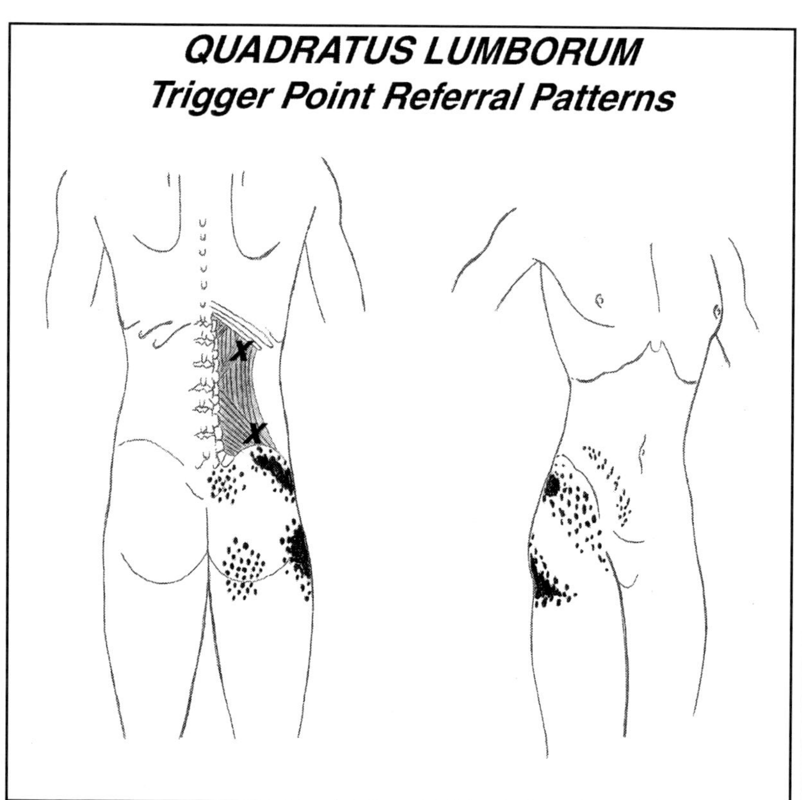

QUADRATUS LUMBORUM
Trigger Point Referral Patterns

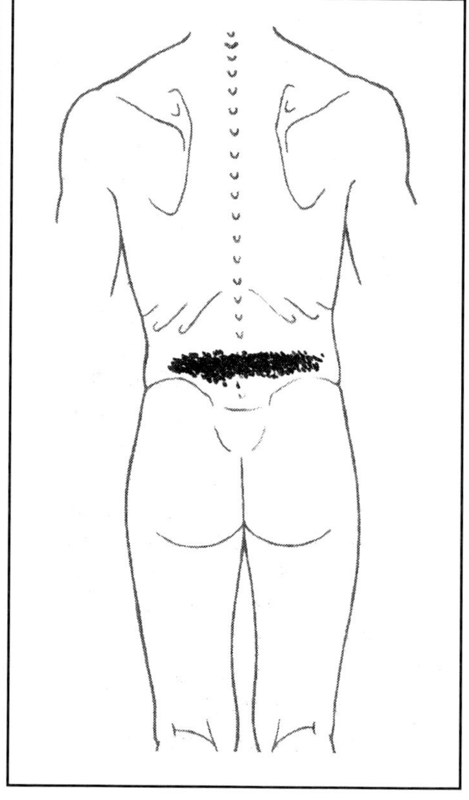

Of course, posture is the biggest culprit. But often the client is valiantly trying to imp his posture, but twisted, tangled, locked short, locked long, or snarly muscles preven him. Another cause, as with any other stabilizing muscle, is ligaments that have weakened with age and/or injury. As we age, the quadratus lumborum gets recruited to stabilize even more, leaving it prone to injury.

Because of its attachment at the 12th rib, the quadratus lumborum plays a vital role in respiration. Keep in mind that the iliopsoas has an attachment right next door at T12. If the iliopsoas is locked short near its T12 attachment, it pulls down and slightly rotates the spine away from that side (contralaterally), producing an additional load on the quadratus lumborum, which is trying mightily to stabilize that 12th rib. I've often found that this 12th rib attachment can be the most difficult to fully release. Often full of scar tissue, it has lost its suppleness, inhibiting dynamic and responsive movement of the rib case.

AN EMOTIONAL MUSCLE

As infants we go through a series of fascinating neurological changes as we advance through the stages of movement development. Two movements are inherent in each stage: Pushing and reaching. The push must precede and support the reach; otherwise the reach becomes a falling over. For example, when an infant learns to walk, she must push hard down into her little feet before a stable, vertical reach can occur. I think of the quadratus lumborum as a "push" muscle, which translates to qualities such as resourcefulness, stability, confidence, personal power, strength, and how supported we feel both internally and externally.

The quadratus lumborum, like the iliopsoas, is a bridge tissue between the upper and lower body. It can become an emotional and energetic dumping site for our unmet needs, frustrations, anger, and grief around issues of support. It stores energies and emotions that need to flow through the pelvis, down the legs, and out the feet, instead of stagnating in our core. Unloading the quadratus lumborum and the spine by lying on the floor or directly on the Earth not only has bio-mechanical benefits but delivers a powerful kinesthetic message of support: *We can let down into a generous and abundant Mother Earth.*

Remember, the sturdy quadratus lumborum is one of the structures that stabilizes the pelvis and lumbar spine so we can walk. The health of this muscle contributes to our ability to move forward in life with power and ease, both literally and metaphorically. Feeling stuck and trapped in a soul-numbing job or an unfulfilling relationship are two examples of energetic/emotional disturbances that could manifest in a locked quadratus lumborum.

Problems in the quadratus lumborum can also show up when we are offering too much support to others and neglecting ourselves. This hardy muscle has much to do with our personal sense of power. It reveals how good we are at taking care of ourselves in all aspects of our lives, and how often we ask for help when we need it. When we're in the "victim vibe" we collapse and compress our vertebrae. In that situation, the quadratus lumborum shortens, losing its length and its robust flexibility and strength.

PROTOCOLS FOR WORKING THE QUADRATUS LUMBORUM

In this section you'll find:

1. Assessment tests and preliminary corrections
2. Positional Release technique
3. Prone, side-lying and supine protocols for releasing the quadratus lumborum
4. Active movement suggestions for Muscle Swimming
5. Working the quadratus lumborum with tools
6. Table stretches

Contraindications for working the Quadratus Lumborum

1. The quadratus lumborum is the somatic voice of the kidneys: kidney pain manifests as low back pain except it is a much deeper non-muscular ache. If you suspect kidney pain, refer to a doctor immediately.

2. If your client has a history of trauma (abuse of any kind, rape, torture, etc.) approach this work with caution. If you do not feel comfortable bearing witness to the intense emotions that may arise, please refer to a psychotherapist or a body/mind therapist.

Assessment Tests

Assessment tests are useful guidelines that along with postural observations, gait assessment, pain patterns and palpation can give us a global picture to keep in mind as we work locally. I've included the following assessment test which I perform before and after the deep tissue/trigger point and stretching protocols:

1. Test for a short quadratus lumborum (high ilium/hip).
2. Preliminary corrections for short quadratus lumborum
3. Also included is a simple positional release technique for a short quadratus lumborum. I've found that doing this easy procedure along with the preliminary correction prepares the muscles for the deep tissue/trigger point protocols.

TEST 1: Test for short quadratus lumborum (high ilium)

When muscles exert an unbalanced force on the pelvis, they can cause one iliac crest to be pulled higher than its counterpart. The quadratus lumborum is intimately involved in this syndrome, which can and does cause a kinetic chain reaction throughout the body, including functional short leg syndrome which studies[2] have found contributes significantly to low back pain.

Client is standing. Therapist kneels behind client.

Step 1: Place the lateral edge of your thumbs horizontally into the soft tissues in the lumbar region, just above the iliac crests. Press in and down until you have contacted the most superior aspect of the ilium. Make sure your point of contact is equidistant from the spinous processes (approximately 1 - 1.5 inches lateral to the spinous processes).

Step 2: Lean back until your elbows are extended.

Step 3: Determine which side is short. **Work and stretch the short side first**. Always work both sides, although one side will usually require more attention.

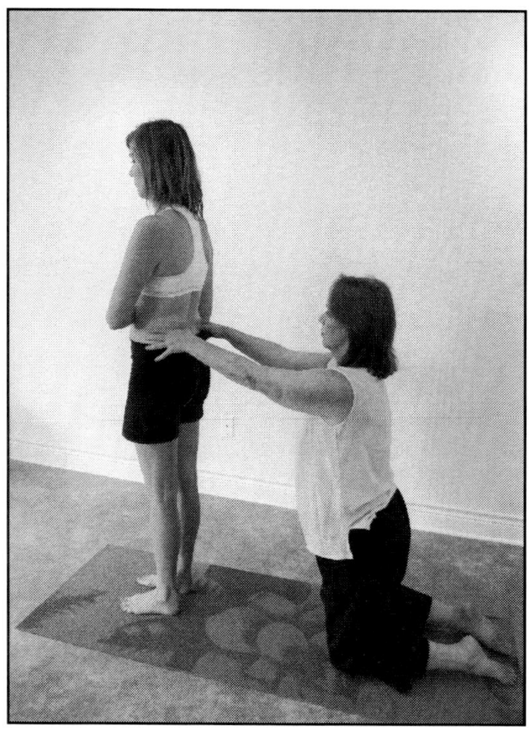

Left: Steps 1 and 2

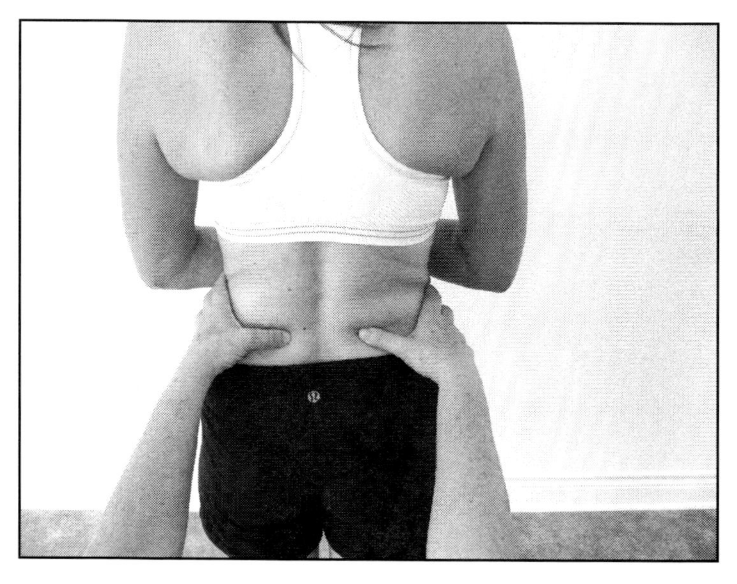

This person's right hip is slightly higher than her left.

[2]*Denslow J, Chase I, et al. Mechanical stresses in the human lumbar spine and pelvis. Postural Balance and Imbalance. Peterson B, ed. Indianapolis: American Academy of Osteopathy, 1983, pp. 76-82.*

Preliminary correction for short quadratus lumborum (high ilium)

Think of this maneuver as a gentle re-positioning of the bones rather than a stretch.

Client is side-lying with the high ilium on the table.

Step 1: Place your uphill hand on the lateral aspect of the iliac crest. Gently traction the crest toward the feet while you also exert a moderate posterior push on the same crest. In other words, the hand that's on the iliac crest is gently pushing in two directions at the same time: posterior and inferior.

Step 2: Wrap your downhill arm around both ankles and lift the lower legs off the table and gently pull them towards the client's head. The knees and thighs remain on the table.

Step 3: Instruct client to take a deep breath, hold it, and gently (5-10% of effort) push her feet down toward the massage table isometrically as you provide resistance by gently pushing up. Have them hold the contraction for 6-8 seconds, then relax/exhale and repeat 2-3 times. Feel for the slight yielding of the pelvis in a caudal direction.

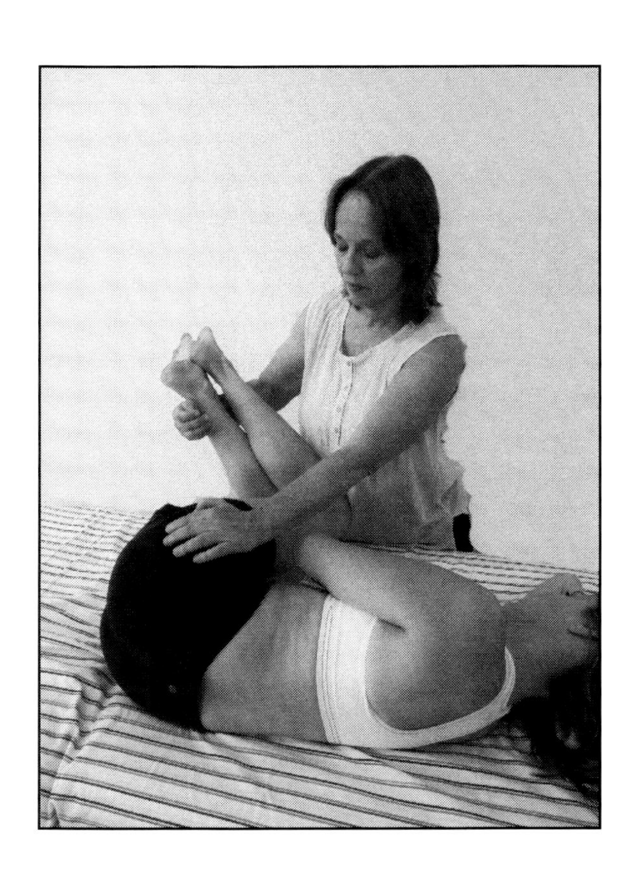

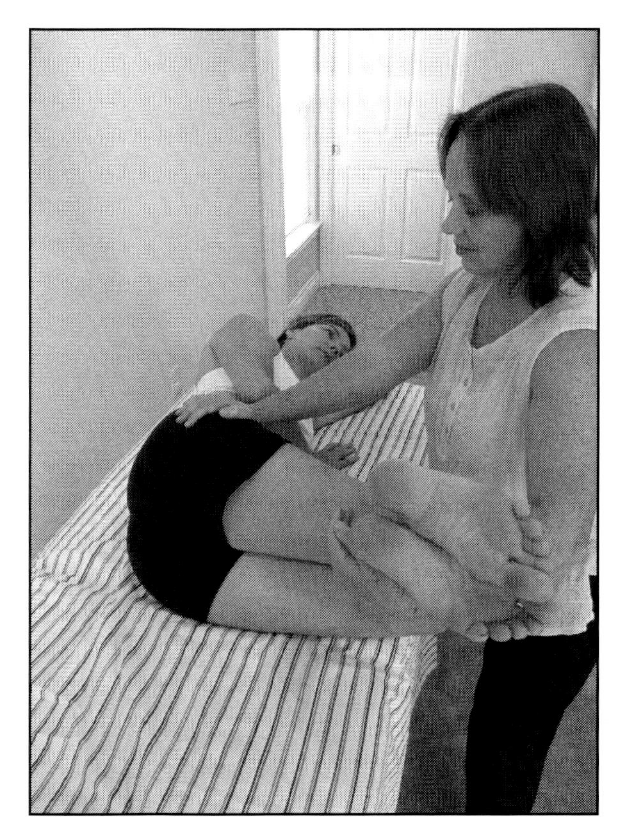

POSITIONAL RELEASE FOR SHORT QUADRATUS LUMBORUM

This is an excellent "pre-release" of the quadratus lumborum which prepares the muscle and the client for deeper work directly on the muscle. I find it to be valuable in creating receptivity in the tissue. The technique is simply to place the muscle in a passive shortened state and hold about one to two minutes.

Client is prone:

Step 1: Maneuver is done on the high ilium side.

Step 2: Downhill hand is on the foot; uphill hand is on the femur.

Step 3: Gently push the leg up toward the head, causing the ilium to "hike", which shortens the quadratus lumborum (see circled area in photo below.)

Step 4: Hold for about two minutes.

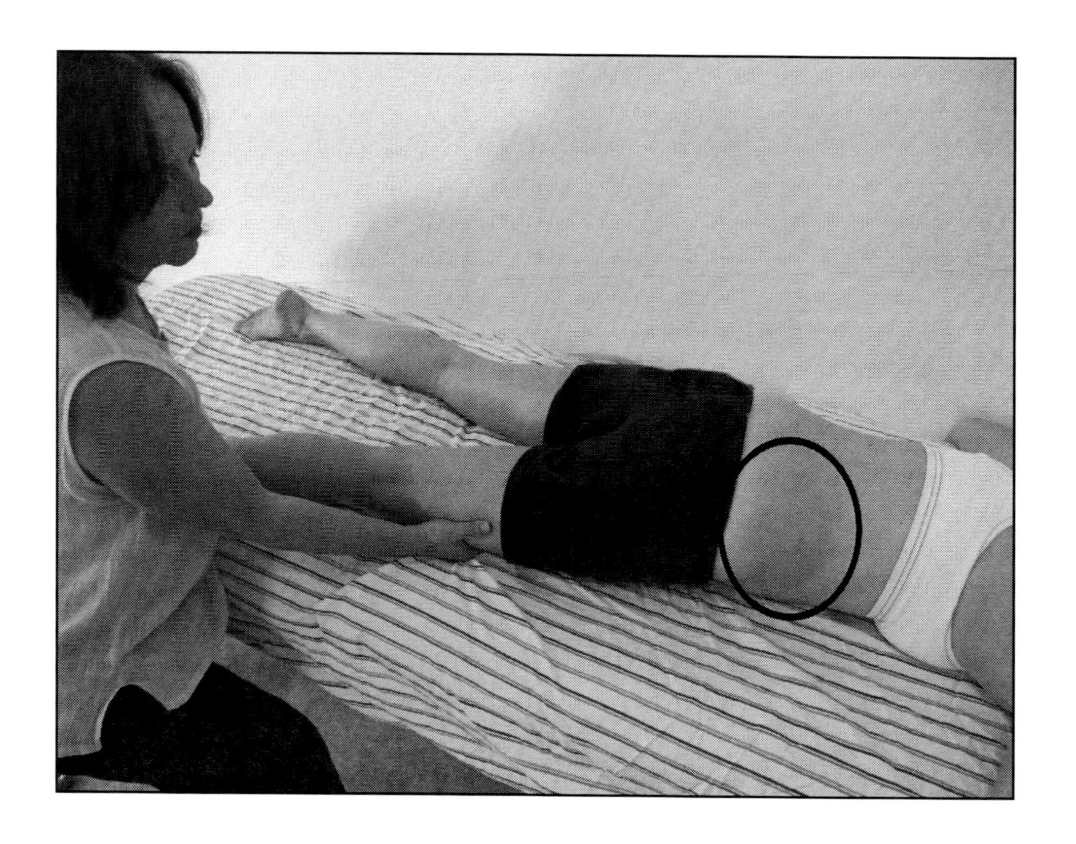

PRONE PROTOCOLS

The quadratus lumborum lies underneath and lateral to the erector spinae. Find the lateral edge of the erector spinae, continue out laterally about a half inch to an inch, then go under the erector spinae and press medially towards the spine. You can verify your location by asking your client to hike the same side hip.

If you've never palpated it on a client, find it on yourself first. In the standing position, place your fingers on your erector spinae on one side. Move your fingers laterally about a half inch to an inch, then go under the erector spinae and press medially towards the spine. Hike the same side hip and you'll feel the substantial QL contract.

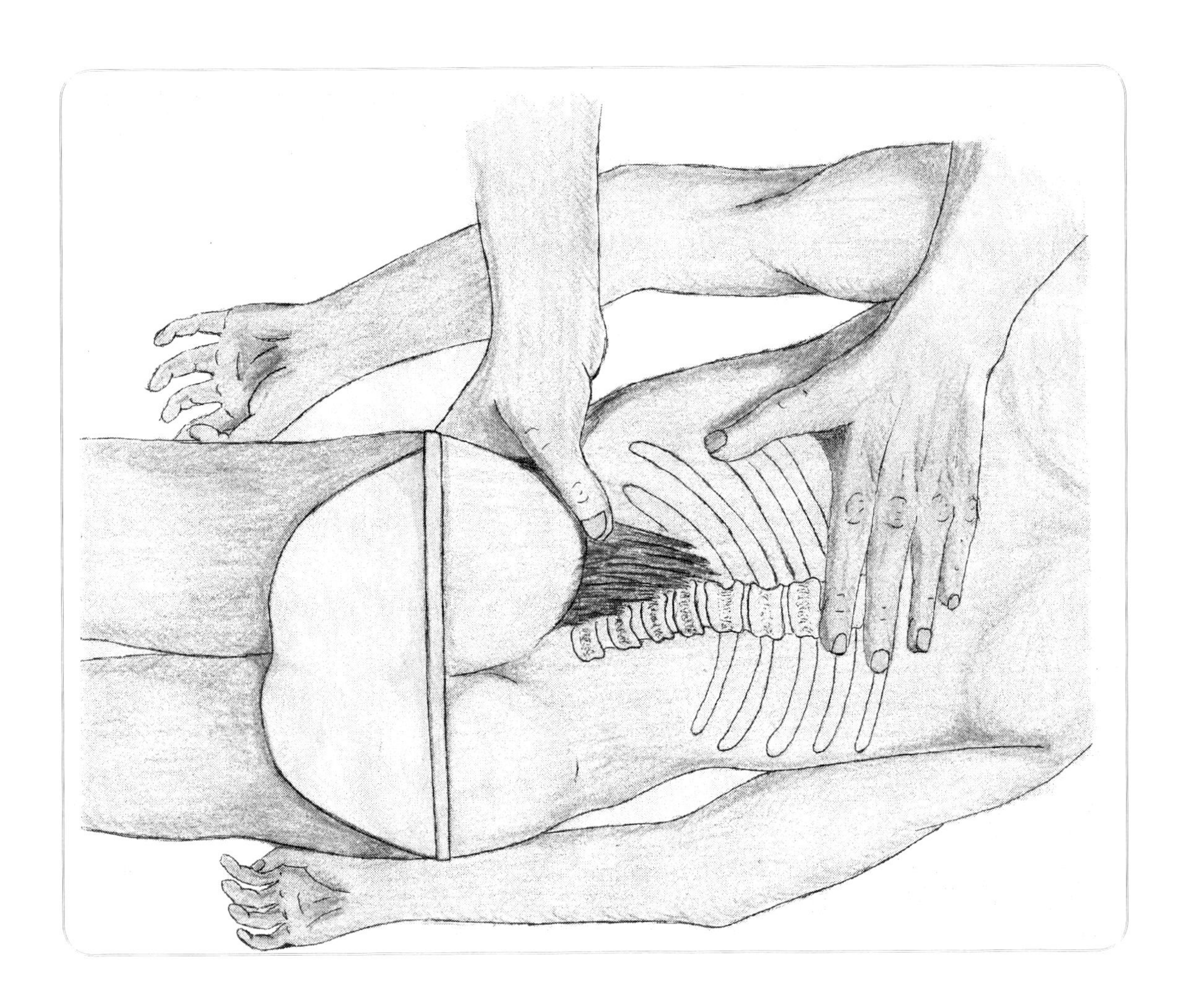

PALPATING THE QUADRATUS LUMBORUM - PRONE

Below: two different approaches to palpating and releasing the QL in the prone position.

In Photo A, the therapist is standing on the same side QL.
In Photo B she is standing on the opposite side of the table.

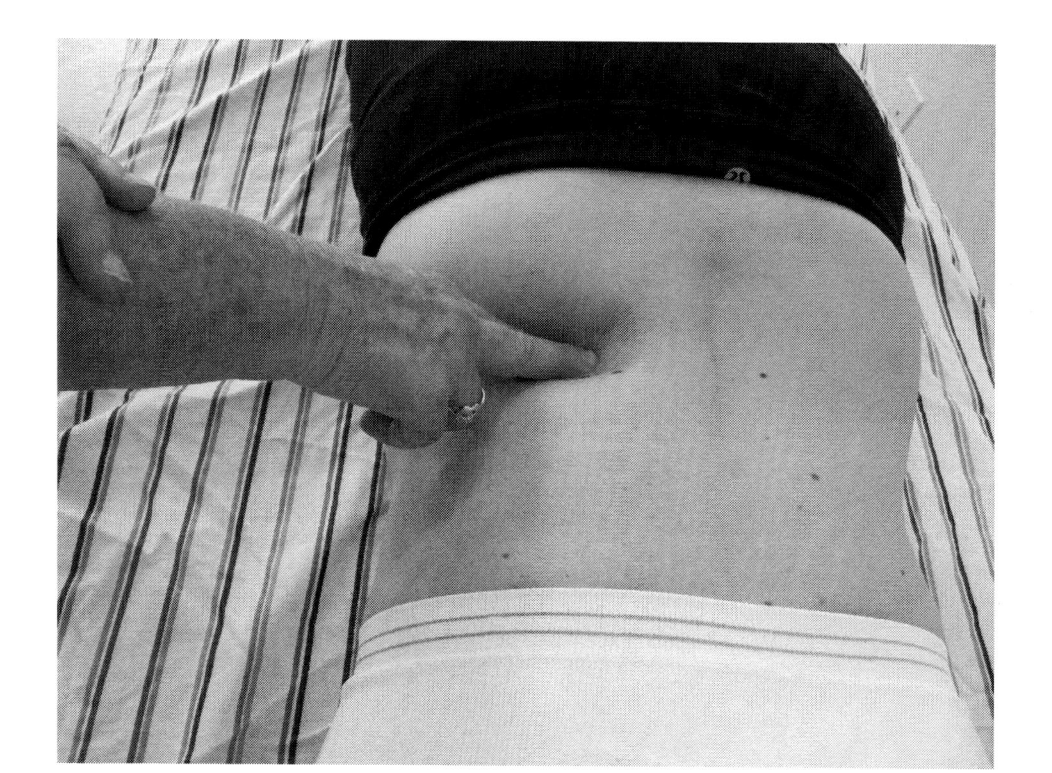

Left: Photo A

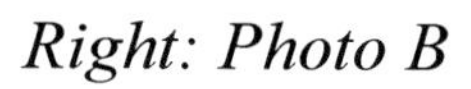

Right: Photo B

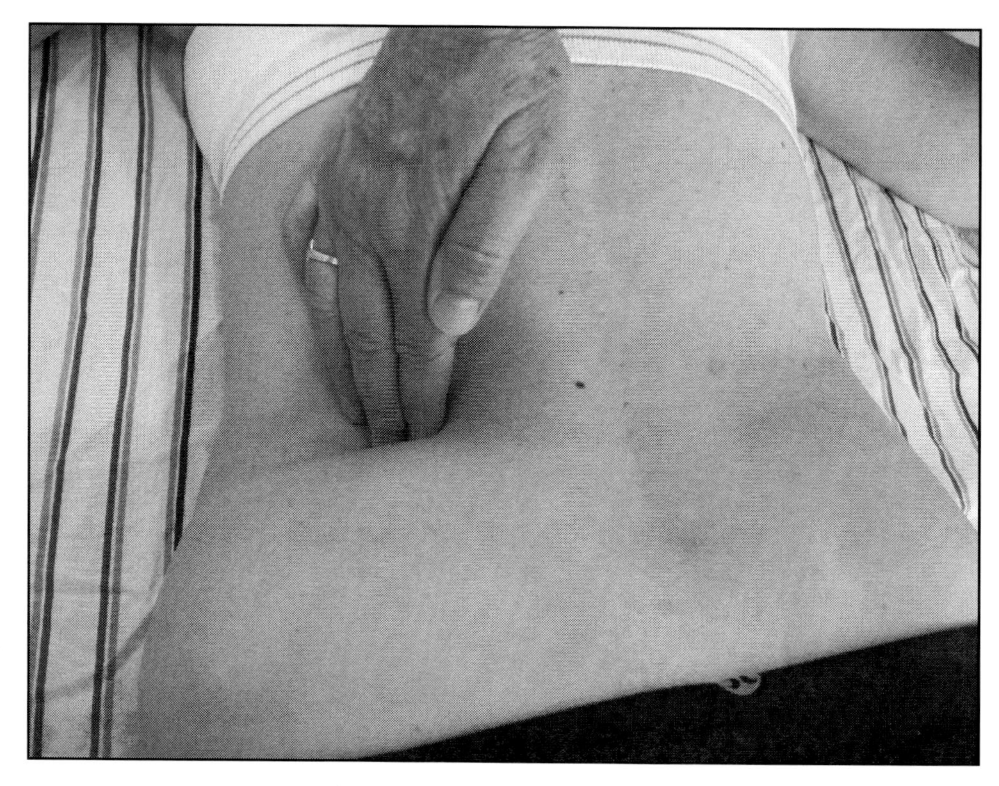

PRONE PROTOCOLS

We'll start our prone work with *skin rolling*. Our goal is to promote healthy superficial fascia. Many factors influence the state of our fascia — nutrition, exercise, hydration, etc. Over time, fascial restrictions and adhesions form, impeding muscle, joint, and ligament function.

Basically, what we are doing here is separating the superficial fascia from the muscles, so that each can do what they are supposed to do without interference from the other.

If you've never skin rolled before, it's easy! Using the pads of your fingers and thumbs, gently pick up a roll of skin at the base of the spine, then simply roll up the spine, always keeping a good roll of skin in your fingers and thumbs. The thumbs push while the fingers gather the skin and pull.

Skin rolling should be multi-directional, since collagen and elastin fibers are multi-directional. Another way of saying that is you can and should skin roll from many directions and angles. Up and down, side to side, diagonally, etc.

STEP 1:

Skin roll the entire back with special attention to the QL.

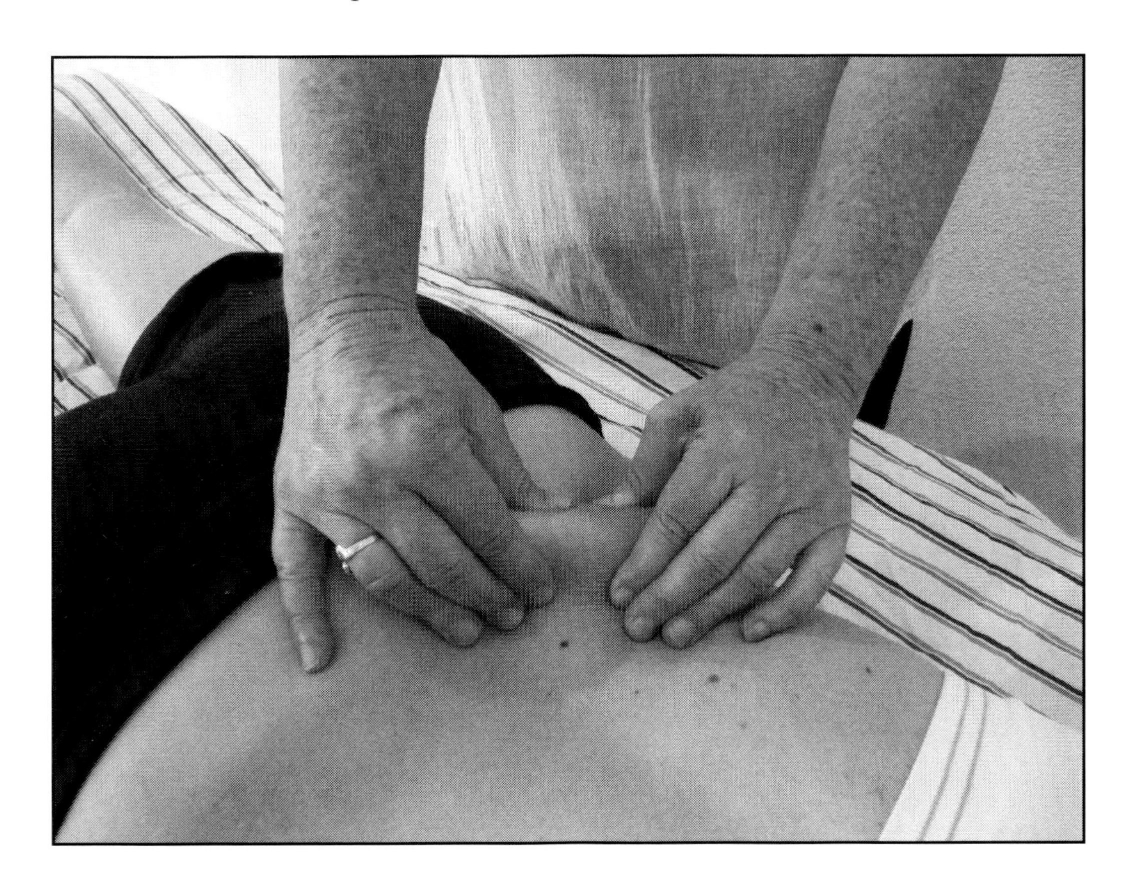

STEP 2 - Warming the tissue:

A. Do some broad gliding (effleurage) strokes over the entire spine.

B. Before we do specific work on the QL, we'll put the muscle in a shortened state just like we did with the positional release technique. Shortening the muscle is the least invasive and usually the least painful way to first approach a muscle.

C. Using finger pads do specific gliding strokes over the QL, gradually increasing the depth of your pressure as the tissue warms. You can do this from the same side or the opposite side. This is a broad warm-up stroke, so use either five or ten fingers, depending on your client's size.

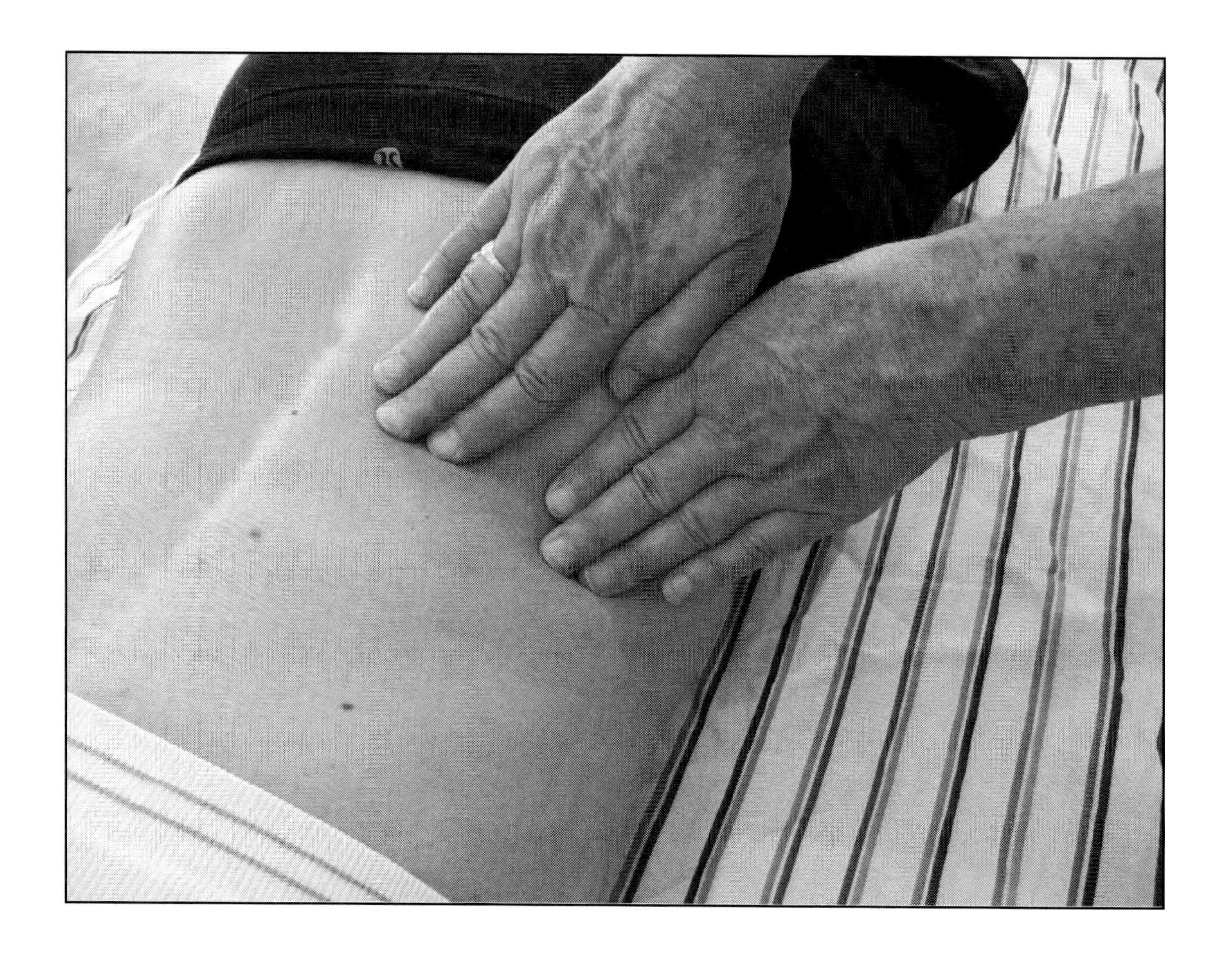

Photo above: Gliding strokes over the QL using the finger pads

PRONE PROTOCOLS

STEP 3 - Assessing the tissue:

Now we'll get more specific and go to one digit or tool. Assess the muscle for tender spots and congested tissue — think of tangled strands of spaghetti. We'll do our trigger point work in side-lying where there are more movement options.

You can incorporate this prone work in your Swedish/relaxation massages. Almost everyone needs QL work!

Below: Feeling for tender spots and congested areas using one finger, thumb, or tool.

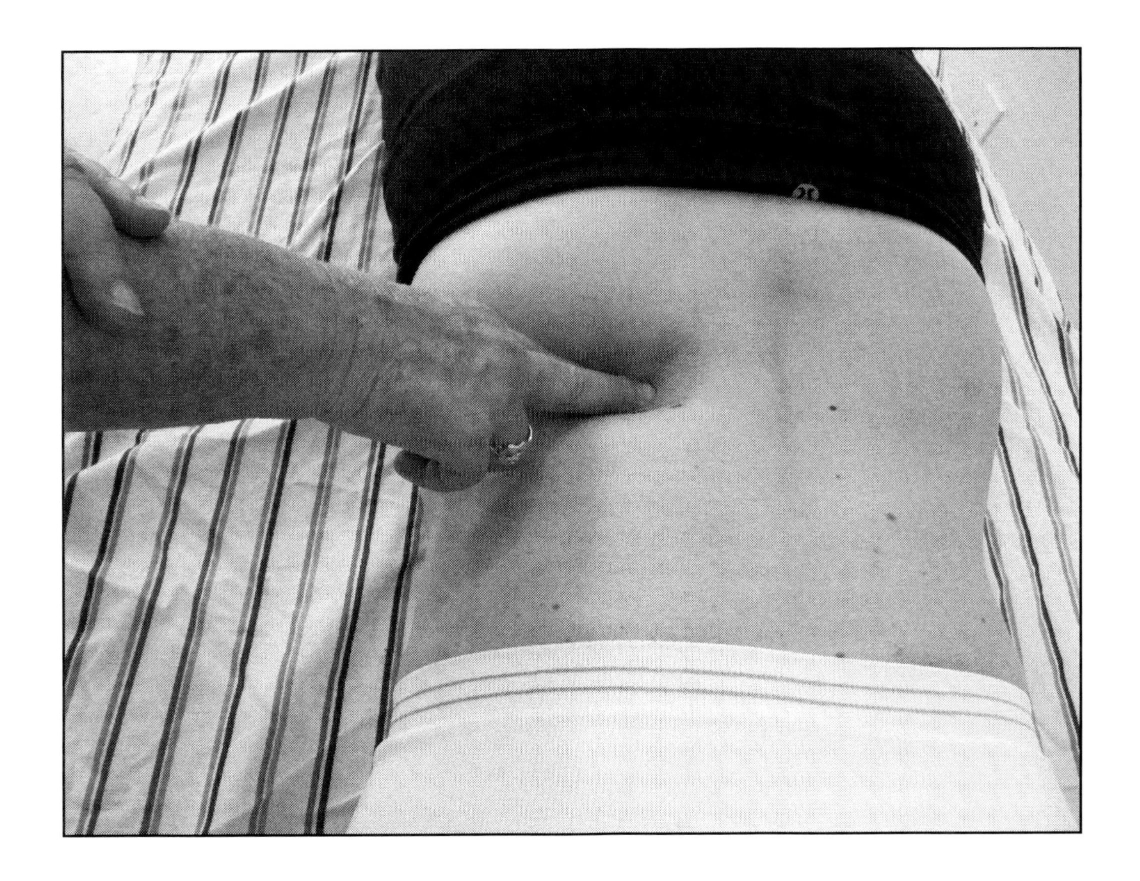

*Reminder: When you find an exquisitely tender spot or trigger point, work to release the tissue **around** it before concentrating on the tender point.*

PALPATING THE QUADRATUS LUMBORUM - SIDE-LYING

The side-lying position offers the most advantages for precise deep tissue work on the quadratus lumborum. This position allows us to work the complex fiber arrangement of the QL with more accuracy. In addition, there are more movement options available so we can Muscle Swim through the layers of the sturdy quadratus lumborum.

If time is an issue, skip the prone protocols and go directly to the side-lying protocols.

Place a small hand towel under the client's waist — this creates more room for deep tissue work. If possible, place the client's top arm behind her head on the table which elevates the thoracic cage, again allowing more space for you to work. If your client's shoulder won't tolerate that position, place that arm on the table and support it with a pillow. Another pillow should also go between the client's thighs.

Find the iliac crest and the 12th rib, then place your fingers halfway between those bony landmarks. Move your fingers about 1/4 to 1/2 inch posterior and gently press toward the table. You will be on the most lateral layer of the QL. Have your client hike her hip to verify your position. You should feel the robust QL shorten under your fingers. Keep in mind you should be pressing deep to the paraspinals.

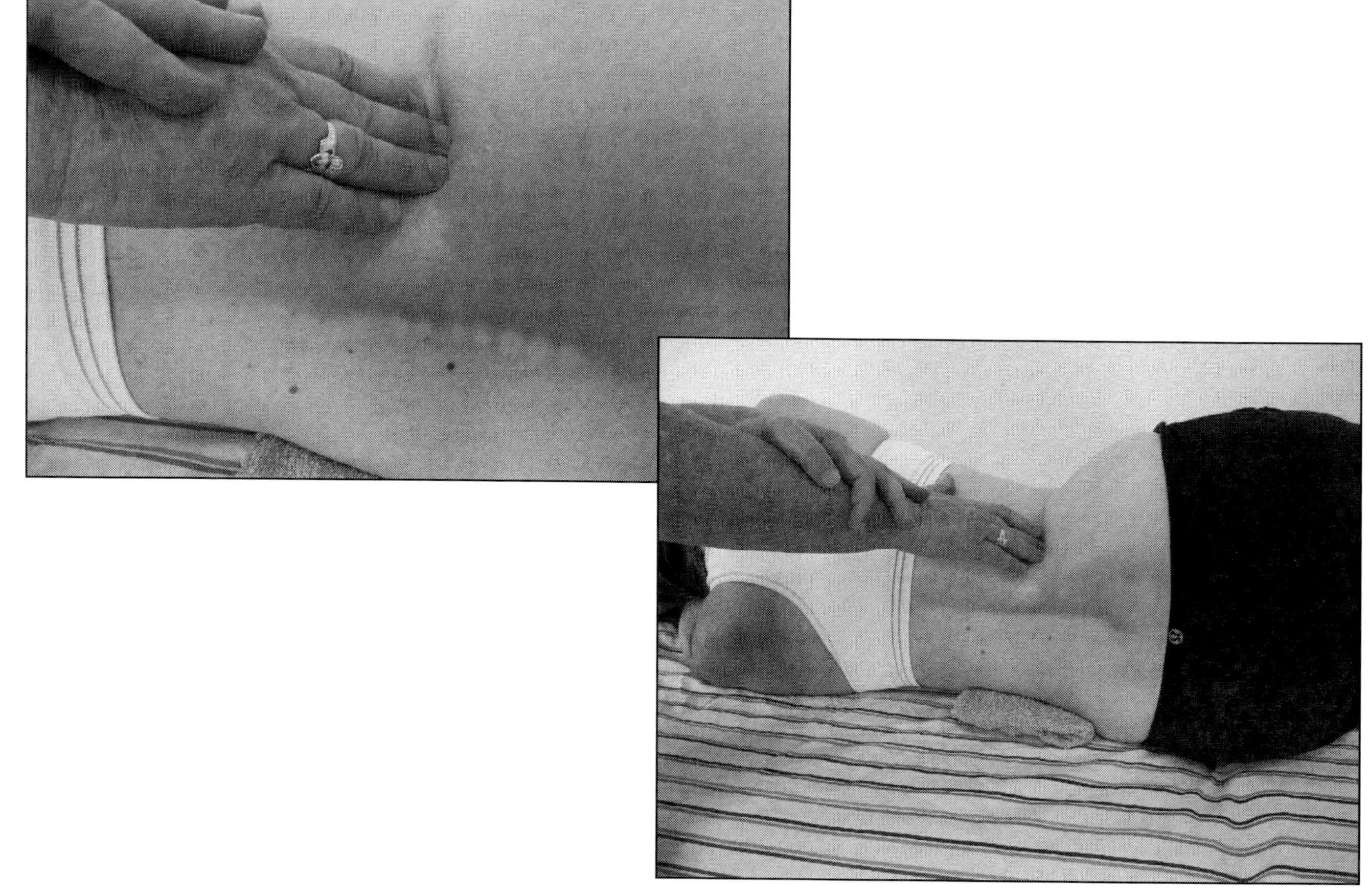

STEP 1:
We'll start with some gentle fascial lengthening. However, if you have not skin rolled the back with special attention to the QL, please do so before this fascial lengthening.

Place your hands crosswise with your uphill hand on the ribs and your downhill hand on the iliac crest. With moderate pressure separate those areas as your client takes several deep breaths. This is a beneficial way to begin our deeper work on the QL. You can and should do this maneuver several times during a session. It can serve as a welcome relief to your client; it's way to give them a break from the more painful trigger point work.

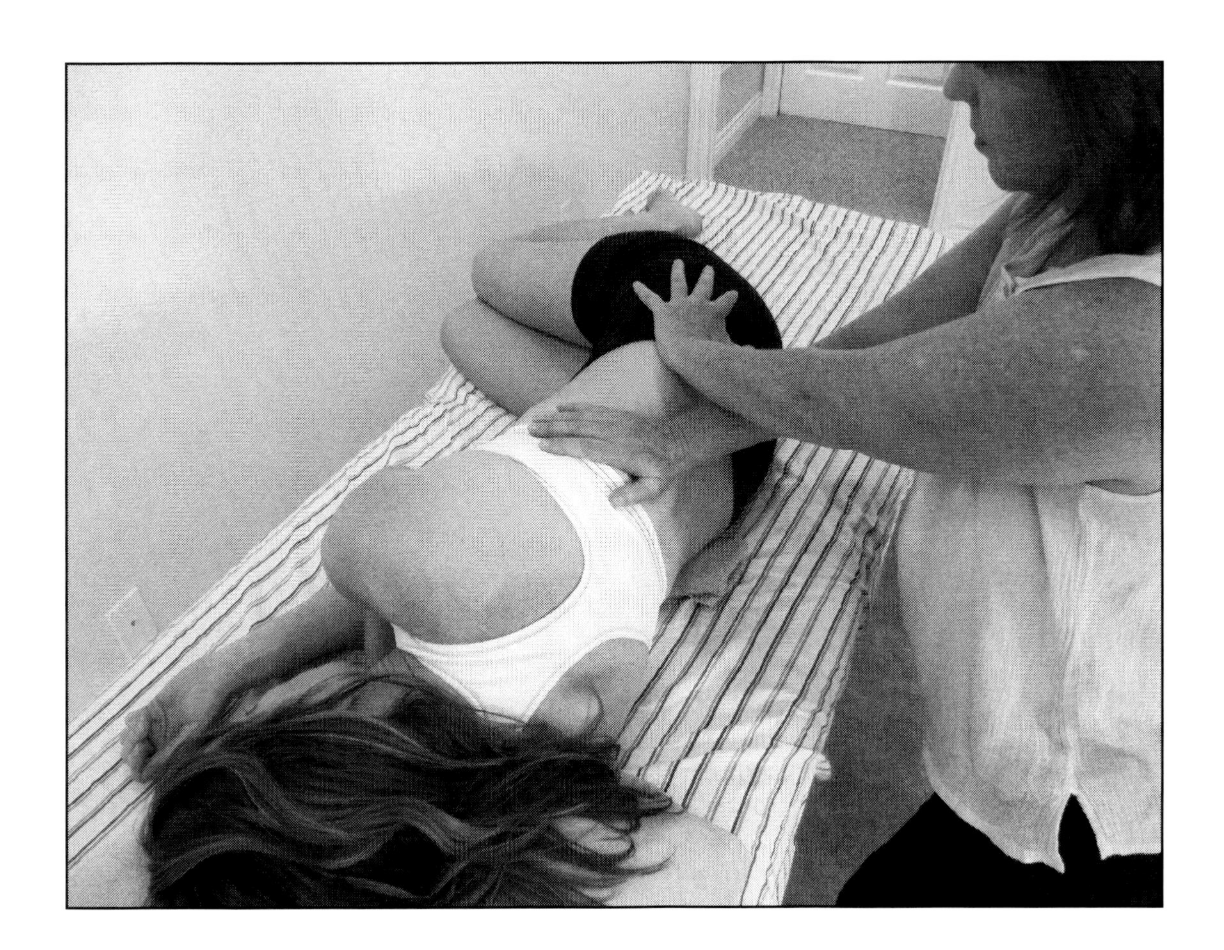

SIDE-LYING PROTOCOLS - Warming the Tissue

STEP 2:

A. We'll use the *Pin and Rock* technique as our way of preparing the QL for deeper work.

Place two or three fingers of your uphill hand on the belly of the QL using gentle pressure. Place your downhill hand on your client's hip. Maintain the moderate pressure on the QL as you slowly rock your client's hips forward and back. Instruct your client to breathe deeply. Do this until you feel the QL begin to soften.

B. After this central part of the quadratus lumborum softens, angle your fingers to the iliac crest and continue this *Pin and Rock* technique. Once you feel that section soften, angle your fingers to the 12th rib and continue this technique. Since we're working in a small area, angling the fingers usually suffices to connect with these attachments.

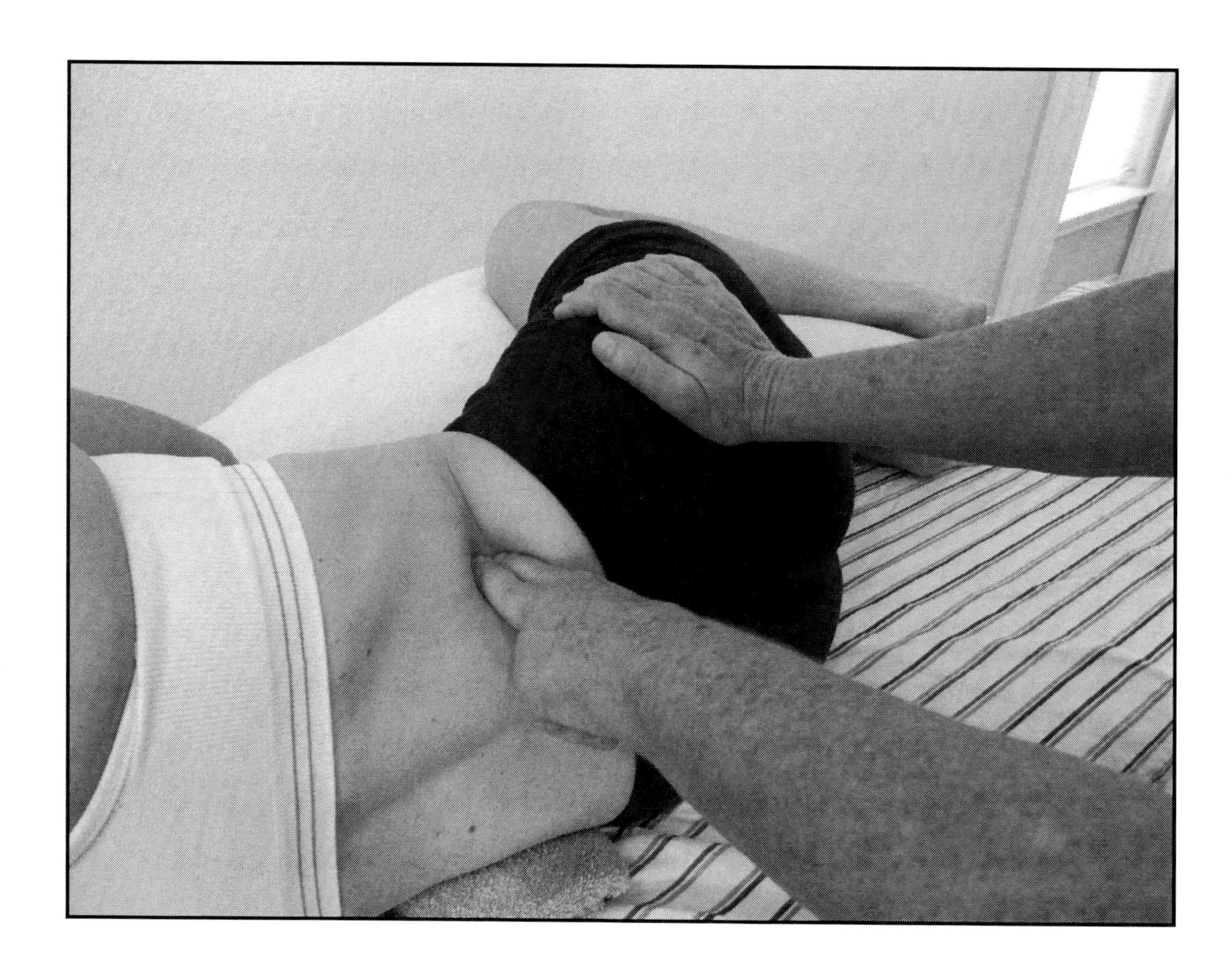

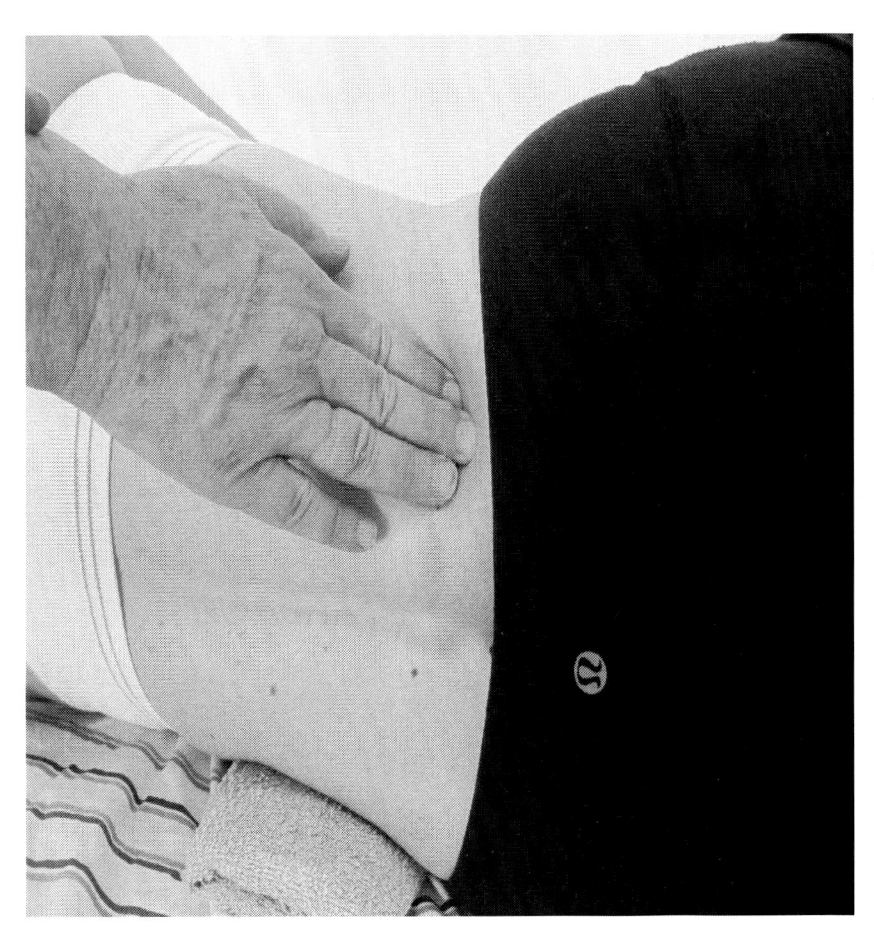

Left: For camera angles, the hand that is rocking the hips was removed to better view the therapist's fingers warming up the attachments at the iliac crest.

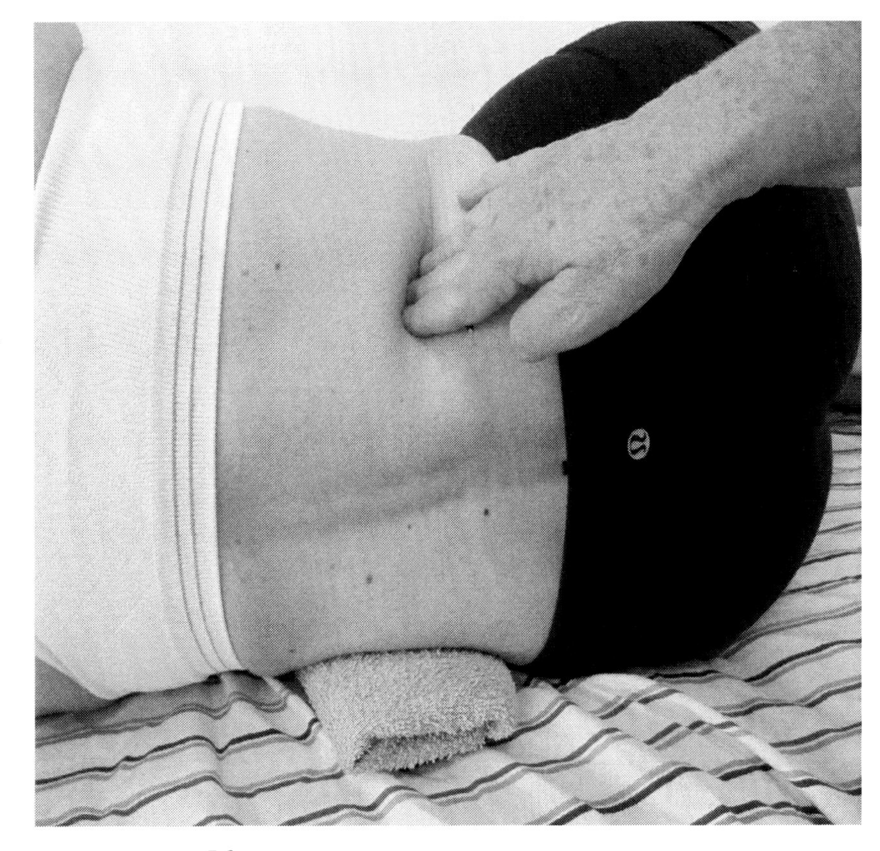

Right: For camera angles, the hand that is rocking the hips was removed to better view the therapist's fingers warming up the attachments at the 12th rib.

SIDE-LYING PROTOCOLS - Warming the Tissue

STEP 3:

After the attachments have softened, return your fingers to the central section of the muscle, continue with the *Pin and Rock* technique, and feel if you can soften and warm up the deeper layers of this powerful muscle where it attaches to lumbar vertebrae 1-4. It's essential that you take the time and patience to warm this area. Many therapists just release the superficial fibers which is good but not good enough!!

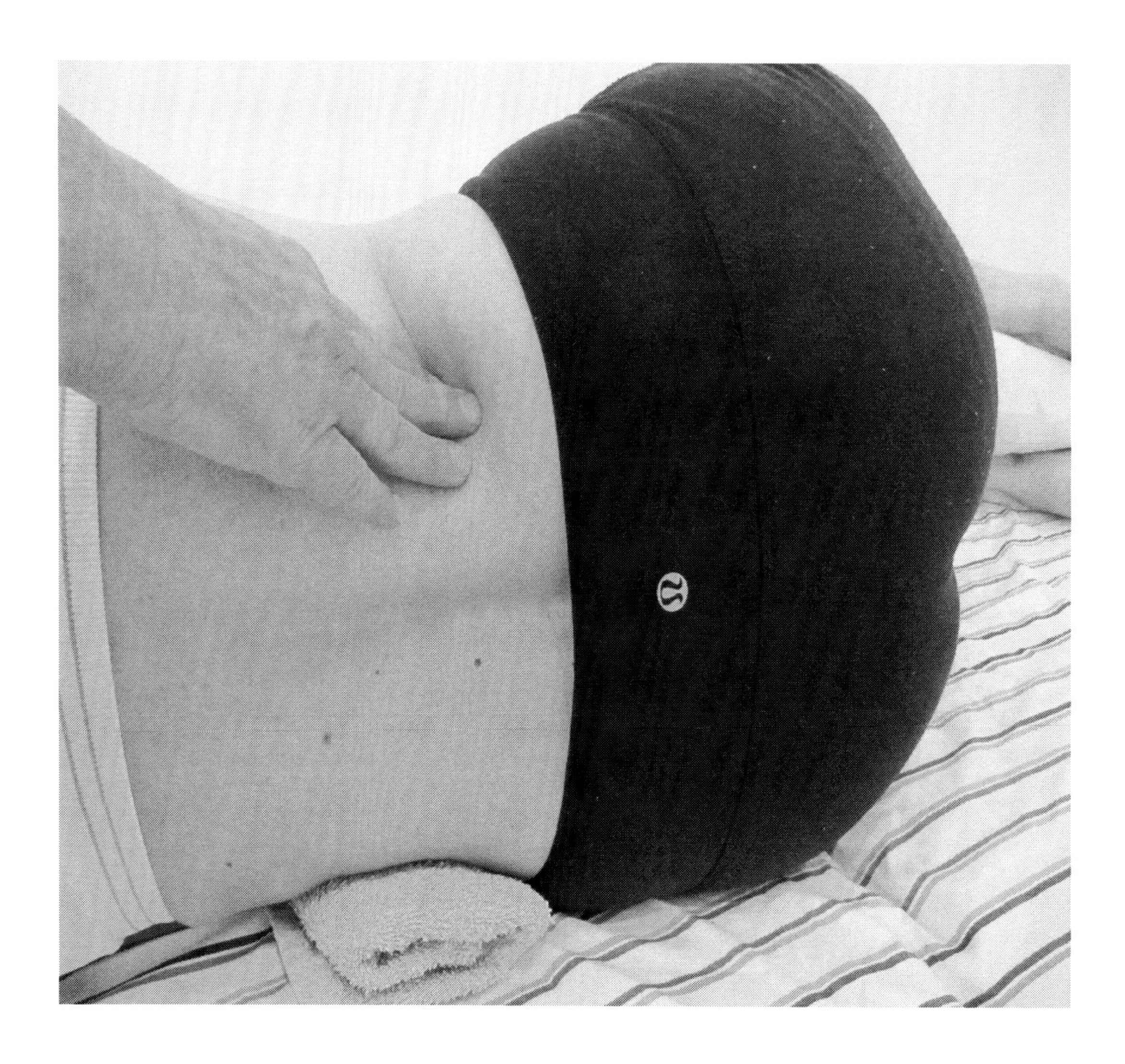

Above: For camera angles, the hand that is rocking the hips was removed to better view the therapist's fingers gently working toward the medial layers of the quadratus lumborum.

SIDE-LYING PROTOCOLS - Going Deeper

STEP 4:
Since the fibers of the QL run in several directions (diagonally and vertically), our next step is to perform a multi-directional fiber stroke in a *6 point system.* We'll work up and down, side to side, and on both diagonals. Think of working in a 6 point star shape.

Do this multi-directional fiber stroke on the belly of the muscle, the attachments at the 12th rib, and the iliac crest.

Make sure not to press directly on the 12th rib but rather hook under it. The QL frequently gets "trapped" there.

When you work the attachment at the iliac crest, hook your fingers under it to thoroughly release the area.

Right: Multi-directional fiber friction on the belly of the QL

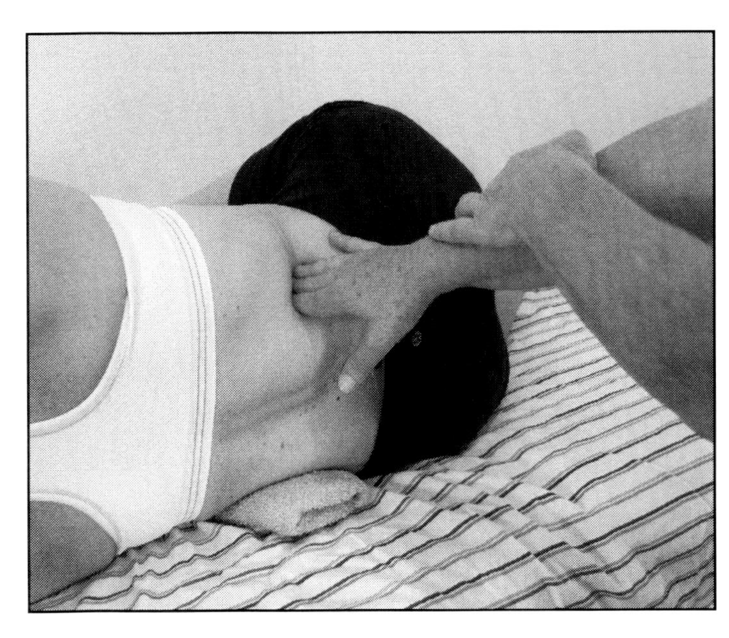

Below left: Multi-directional fiber friction on the iliac crest attachment.

Below right: Multi-directional fiber friction on the 12th rib attachment by hooking under it.

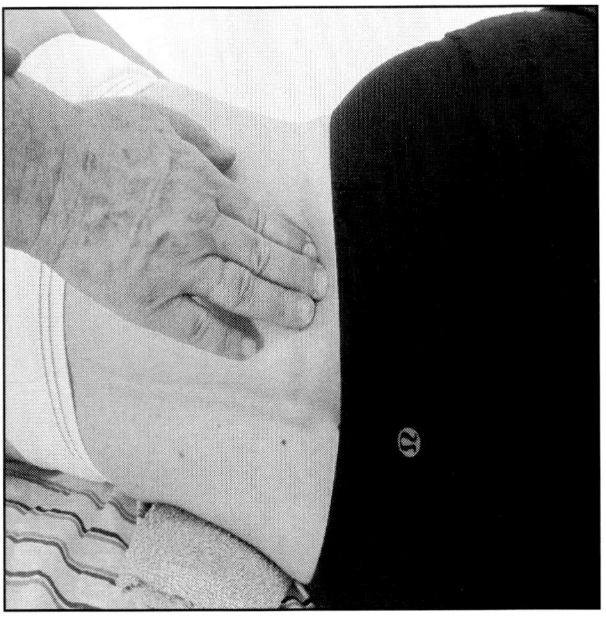

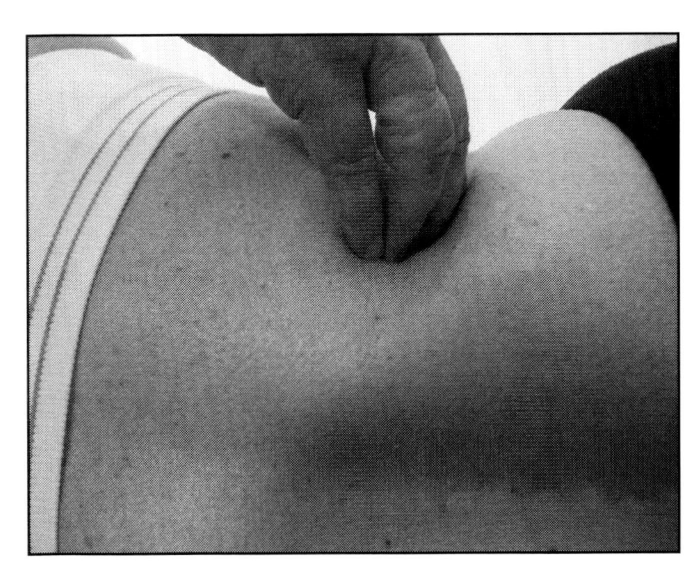

STEP 5:

Once the tissue is warm and receptive, it's time to release knots, adhesions, and trigger points with our *Muscle Swimming with Active Movement*. When you feel a knot, adhesion, or trigger point, gently pin the area while the client does active movement.

A list of possible active movements includes:

A. Thigh flexions/extension.
B. Pelvic tilts.
C. Hip hikes.
D. Lateral flexion of spine.
E. Any combination of the above movements.
F. Adding resistance to any of the above movements. This loads the muscle and recruits more fibers, allowing you to swim through the myofascial tissue.
G. Ask your client if she feels any other movement would be helpful.

You'll see examples of the above movements on the following pages.

A. **Thigh flexions/extensions** are a good place to start. Even though the QL is not directly involved with thigh flexion/extension, the iliac crest shifts during these movements when done in a side-lying position, thereby engaging the QL

I call the maneuver shown on the next page *Running Man*. Teach your client the movement pattern using passive movement and do it for her several times. Then have her do the movement 4-5 times. Check in with her, asking the question, *"Is there any change?"* Using this language instead of *"Is it better?"* gives your client permission to tell the truth.

If she reports that it is better, you'll know the movement pattern is working. If she reports no change, try adding resistance to the pattern. In the case of *Running Man*, this would involve placing your hand on the front of her thigh during the flexion phase and on the back of her thigh during the extension phase.

If adding resistance does not work, try another movement pattern. This is where this work gets interesting; the trial and error of experimenting with different movements and levels of resistance develops our skills and intuition.

TPRpals

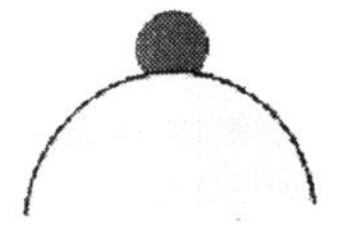

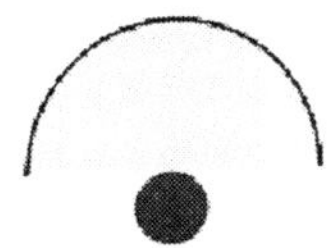

TPRpals are simple, but useful little tools. The intended purpose of the TPRpal is for static, targeted trigger point release by either laying atop them on the floor, table, countertop, leaning into them against a wall, or while sitting in a chair.

1) Insert the wooden knobber tips on round side of the half ball and place the flat side on any flat surface.

2) Locate the tight knotted muscles and slowly let your body weight sink into the wooden knobber tip. It is recommended to remain on a target area for at least 30 seconds. The longer the better. You can slightly oscillate your body upon the tip massaging the immediate area.

3) They can be used as a handlheld massaging knobber (thumbsaver) for deep tissue manipulation on the entire body. Insert the wooden knobber tips on either side of the half ball to accommodate your hand.

Instructions for Running Man

1. Ask the client to slowly slide the top leg towards the chest, keeping the entire leg in contact with the table. The thigh does not need to come into full flexion. Whatever the client can do without straining is fine. The bottom leg should be comfortable with a small degree of flexion at the thigh and knee.

2. Have her slowly slide the top leg into extension

3. Lift that leg about one inch above the bottom leg and place it *behind* the bottom leg.

4. Repeat the above steps 3-5 times while working the tissue.

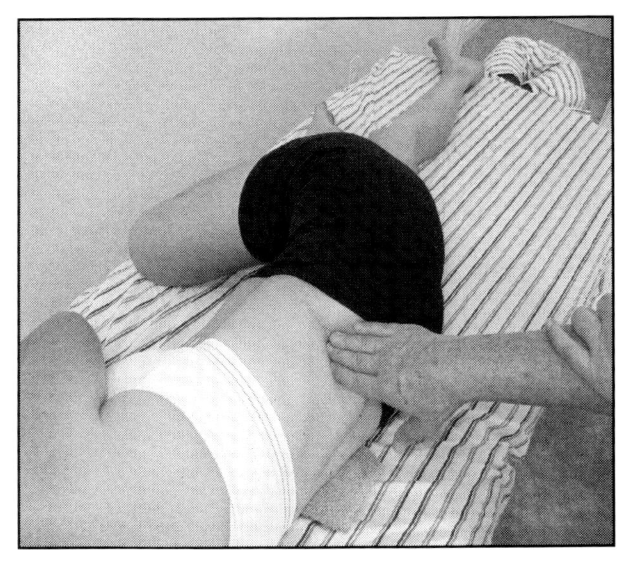

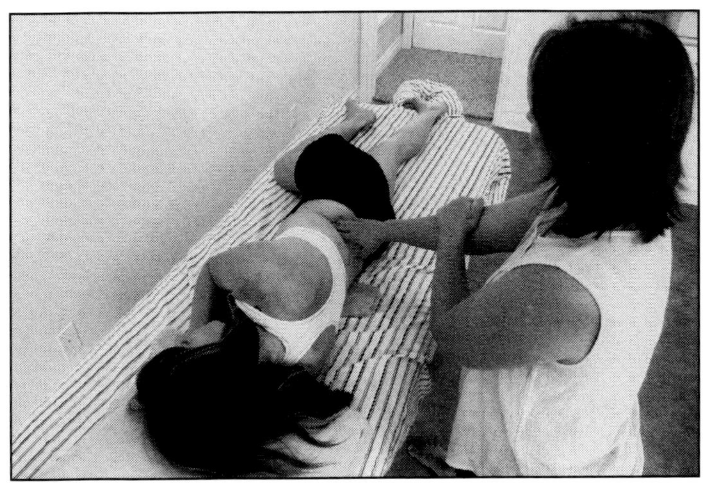

Step One above left: client flexing her thigh

Step Two above right: Client extending her thigh

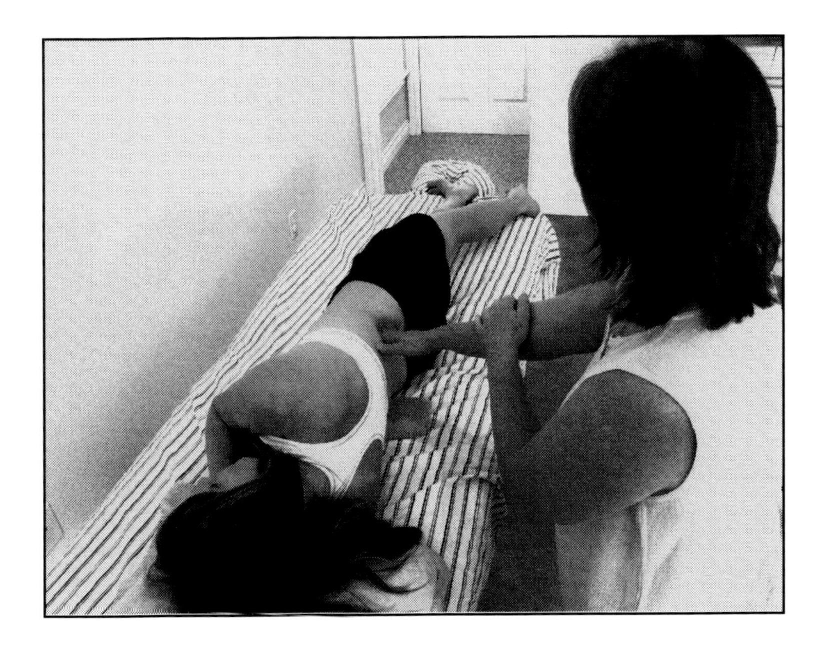

Step Three right: Placing her thigh behind the bottom leg

B. Pelvic tilts (with both knees bent) are also an effective movement pattern to help release stubborn tissue. I call this maneuver *"Good Dog/Bad Dog"*. An easy way to describe this to a client is for her to pretend to be a "bad dog" by tucking the tail bone under in a posterior tilt of the pelvis, and a "good dog", by moving the tail bone up in an anterior tilt of the pelvis. Repeat the above steps 4-5 times while working the tissue.

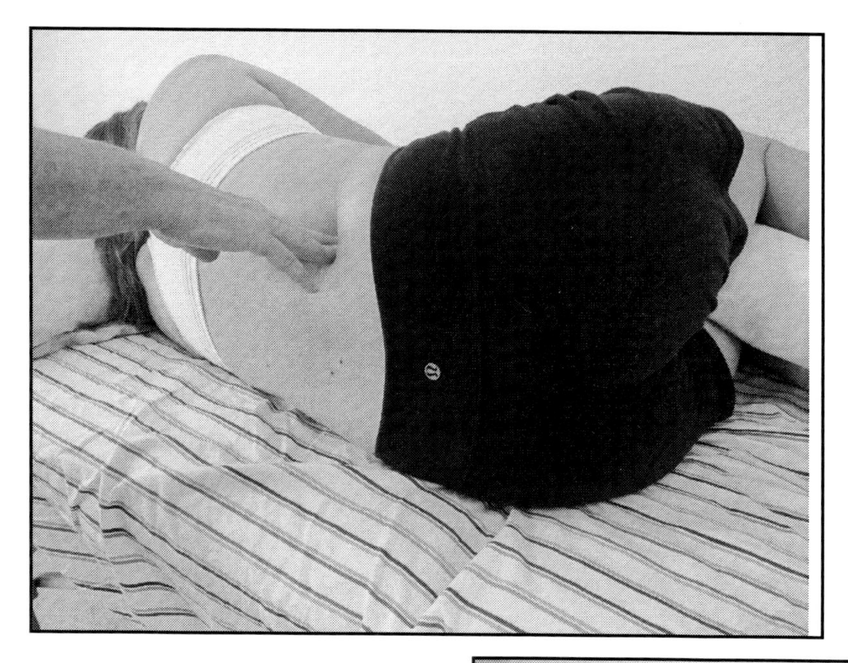

Left: Client tucking her pelvis like a "bad dog" while therapist pins a stubborn section of tissue.

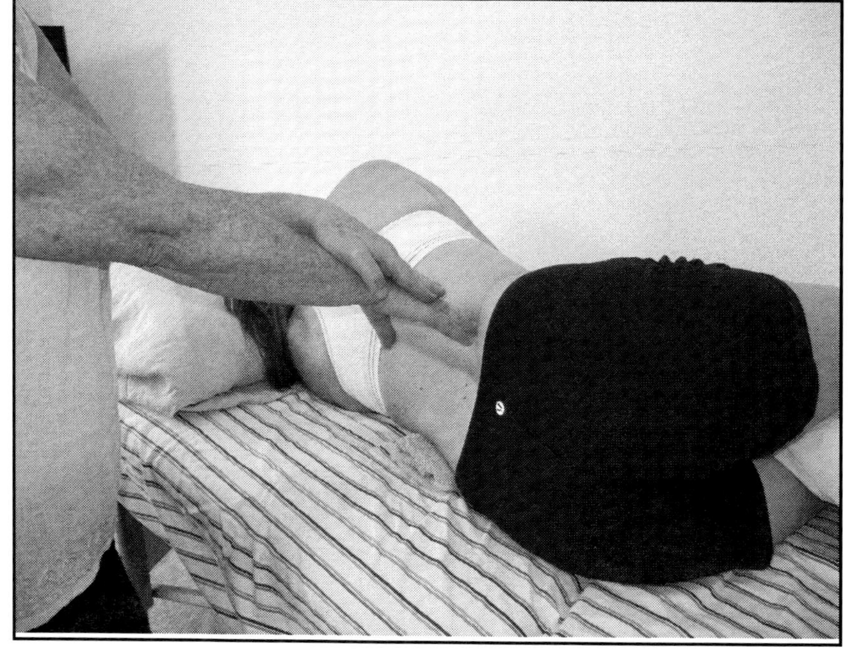

Right: Client tilting her pelvis like a "good dog" while therapist pins a stubborn section of tissue.

Reminder: Keep in mind that slow is better and less is more.

C. Hip Hikes: This movement pattern involves moving the iliac crest toward the ribs. It's a hard one to get for most clients. The easiest way to teach it is for the therapist to do the movement for the client first. Place your downhill hand on the iliac crest and gently move it toward the 12th rib as in Photo A, then away from the 12th rib as in Photo B. Have your client do this movement at least 4-5 timeswhile working the tissue.

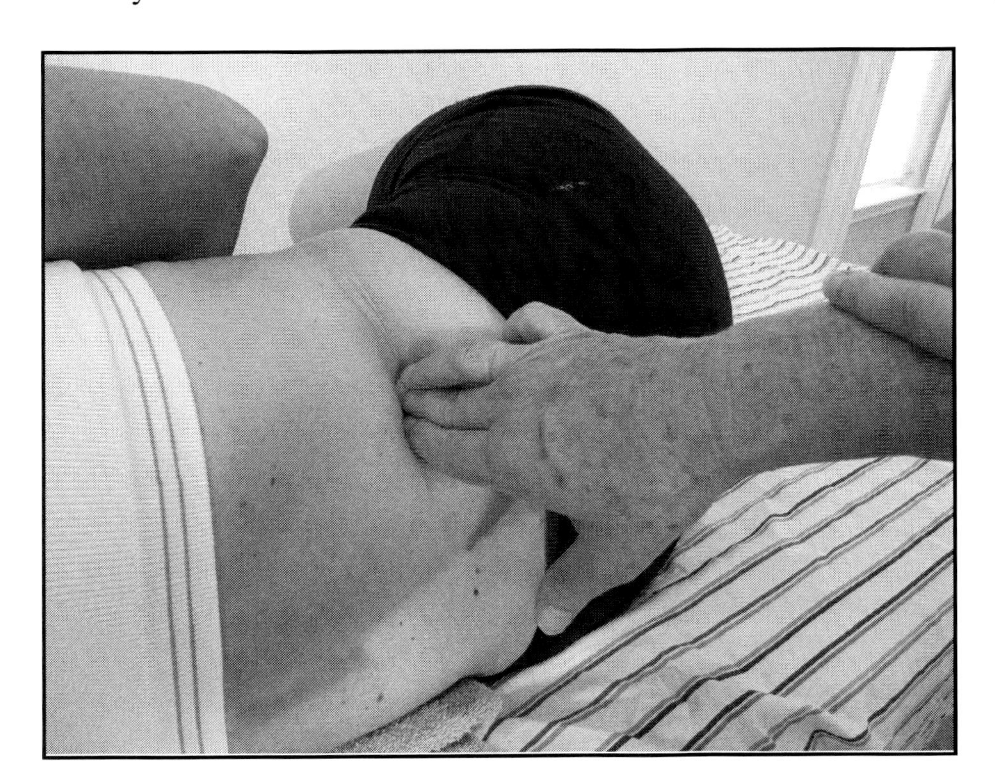

Photo A

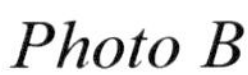

Photo B

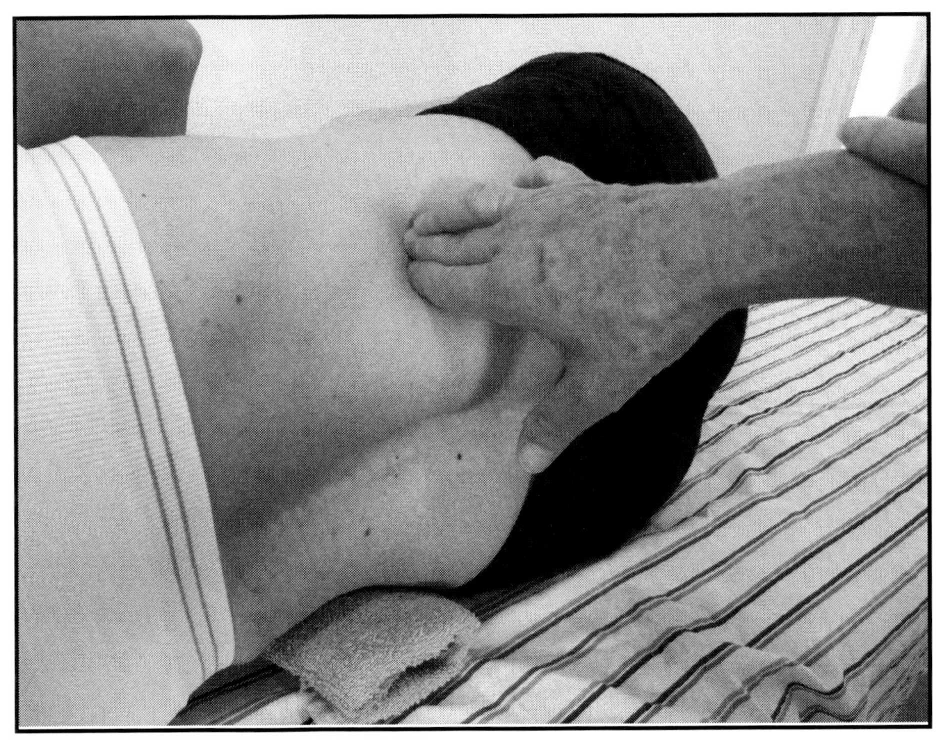

D. Lateral Flexions: Since the quadratus lumborum laterally flexes (side bends) the spine, you also can use this movement to release obstinate tissue. Ask your client to slowly raise her upper body off the table as shown in Photo A, then slowly lower it back to the table as shown in Photo B. This can be a small movement.

Have your client do this movement at least 4-5 times while working the tissue.

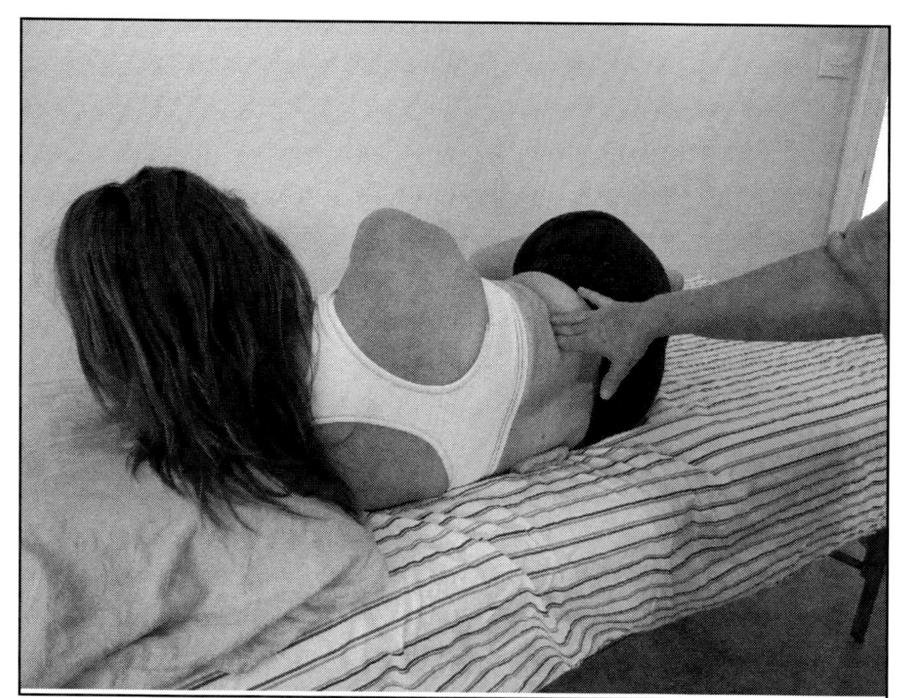

Photo A

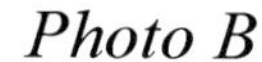

Photo B

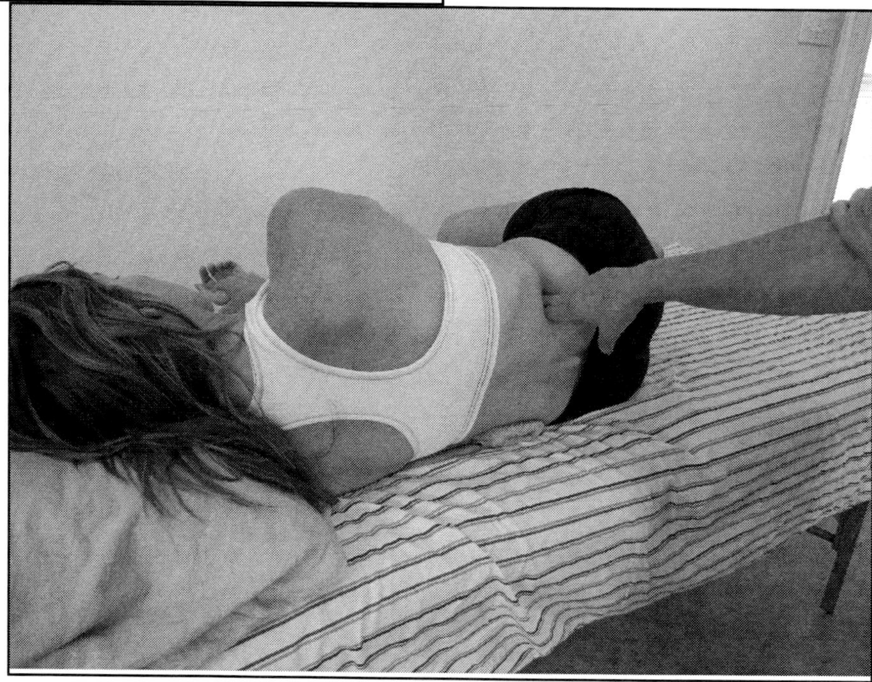

Working the QL with Tools

Working the QL can be tiring on our hard-working hands, and I've found the following tools to be quite handy (pun intended). I especially like the MyoBall and Trigger Point Ball because my clients think I'm using my hands.

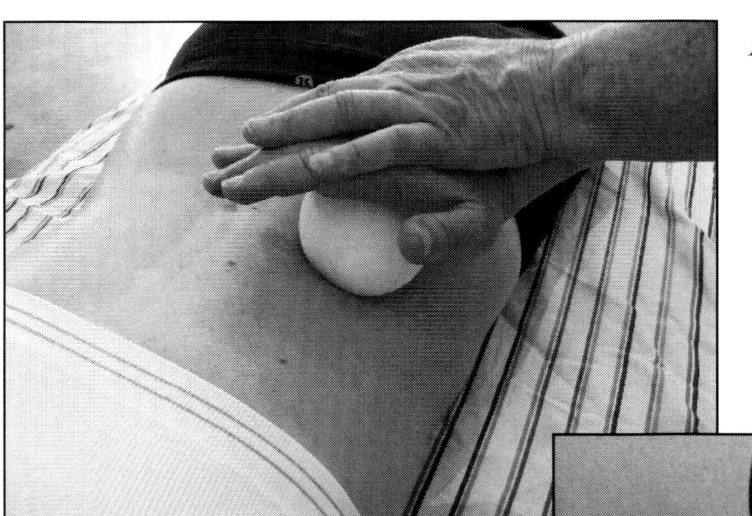

Left: This MyoBall is wonderful for fascial work.

Right: This Trigger Point Ball is just the right size for deep q.l. work and is also wonderful for fascial work.

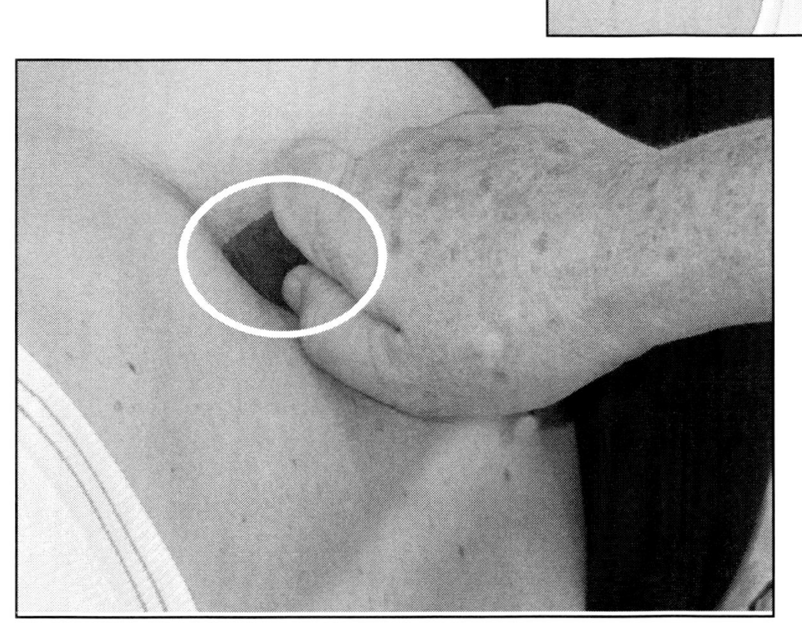

Left: Hot or cold stones are also fabulous for specific trigger point work.

STEP 6: QUADRATUS LUMBORUM STRETCHES

Stretch the high ilium side. Client is side-lying on the side opposite to be stretched and moves her body to the edge of the table. Guide the top leg to hang off the edge of the table. The knee needs to clear the table; sometimes it takes a bit of trial and error to achieve this while maintaining the client's alignment. If you're having trouble getting the knee to clear the table, ask her to scoot her upper body away from you and her rear end towards you. Stabilize the pelvis with your body to prevent rotation or over-arching of the lower back. A pillow under the clients waist can help with positioning and increase the stretch. To use a PNF strategy, have the client push up to engage/shorten the QL, with no more than 20% effort. Client holds the contraction for 8-10 seconds. Therapist then feels if the tissue can stretch farther. Repeat the PNF two more times. PNF techniques are especially good for re-educating the stretch reflex and reducing its signaling on tissue that has an especially short resting length.

Step 1: Gently press down on the femur (less intense) or the calf (more intense) of the leg being stretched with your downhill hand. The client's upper arm must be above the ribs, reaching up towards her head. With your uphill hand traction the iliac crest away from the ribs. Hold for 15-30 seconds.

Step 2: Move your upper hand to the rib case and traction it away from the pelvis, while maintaining the pressure on the femur or calf. Hold for 15-30 seconds.

Step 3: To come out of the stretch, lift the leg back onto the table, so the client does not engage the muscle.

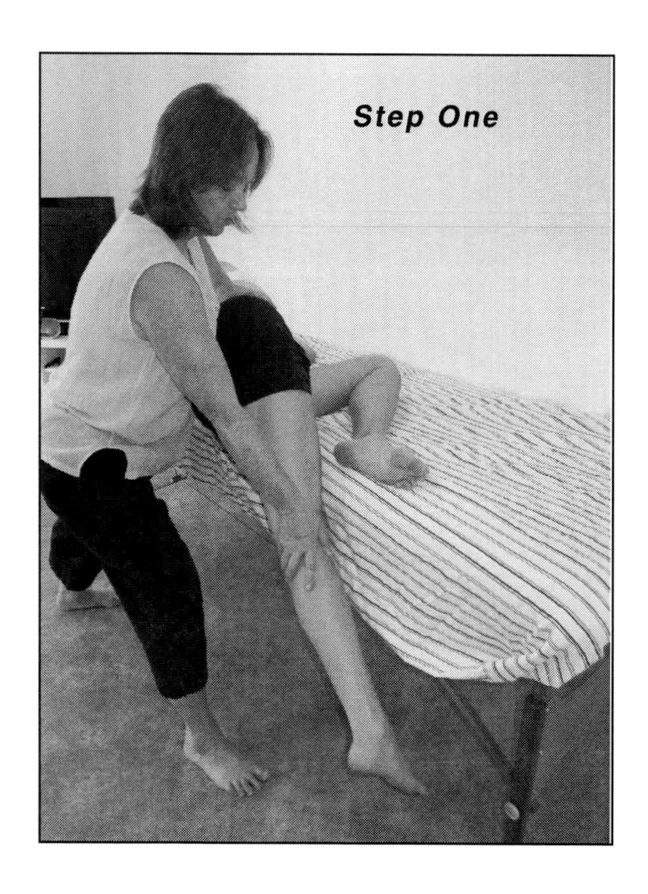

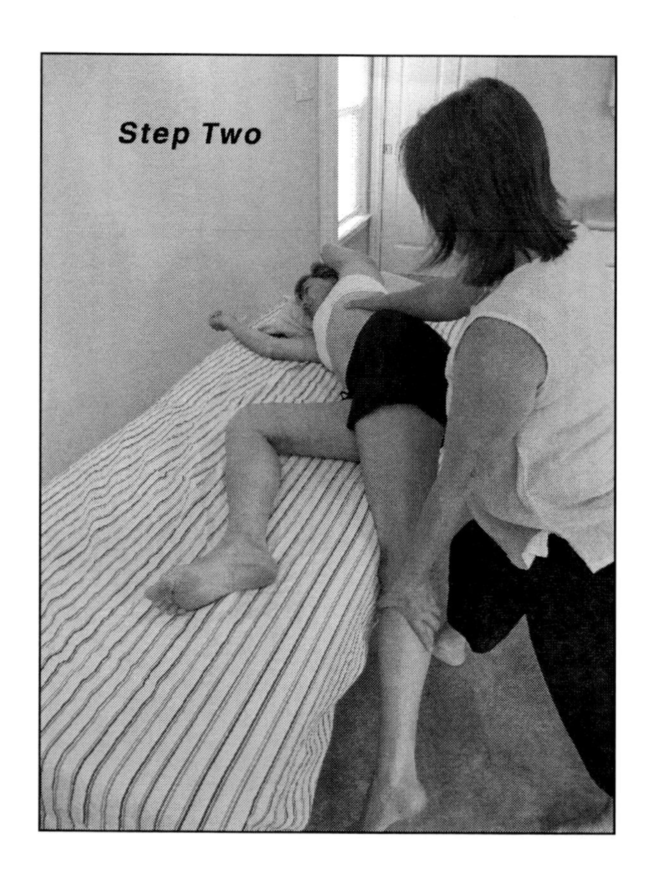

STEP 6: QUADRATUS LUMBORUM STRETCHES

I've found that some clients feel this stretch in their quadratus lumborum more than the preceding stretch while other clients feel very little from this stretch. It's good to know several stretches for a muscle because we're all unique and what works on one client may not work on another.

Client is lying on the side to be stretched, with the lower arm above the ribs.

Step 1: Place your uphill hand on the lateral aspect of the iliac crest. Gently traction the crest toward the feet while you also exert a moderate posterior push on the same crest. In other words, the hand that's on the iliac crest is gently pushing in two directions at the same time: posterior and inferior.

Step 2: Wrap your downhill arm around both ankles then lift the lower legs off the table. Gently pull them towards the client's head. The knees and thighs remain on the table.

Step 3: Hold for 15-30 seconds.

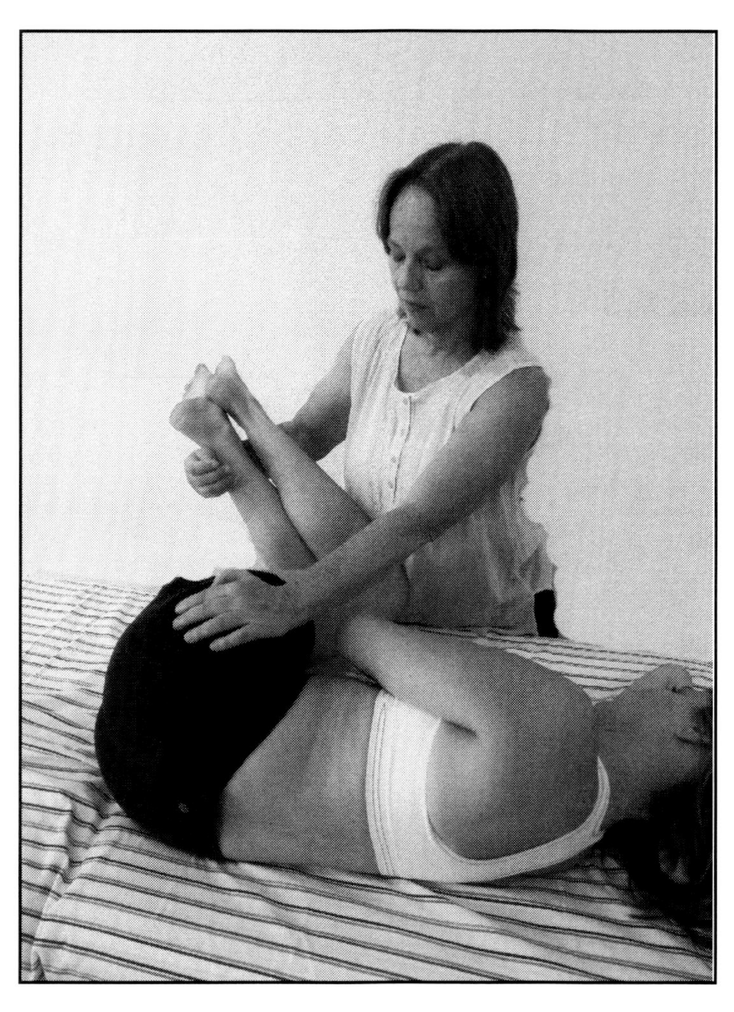

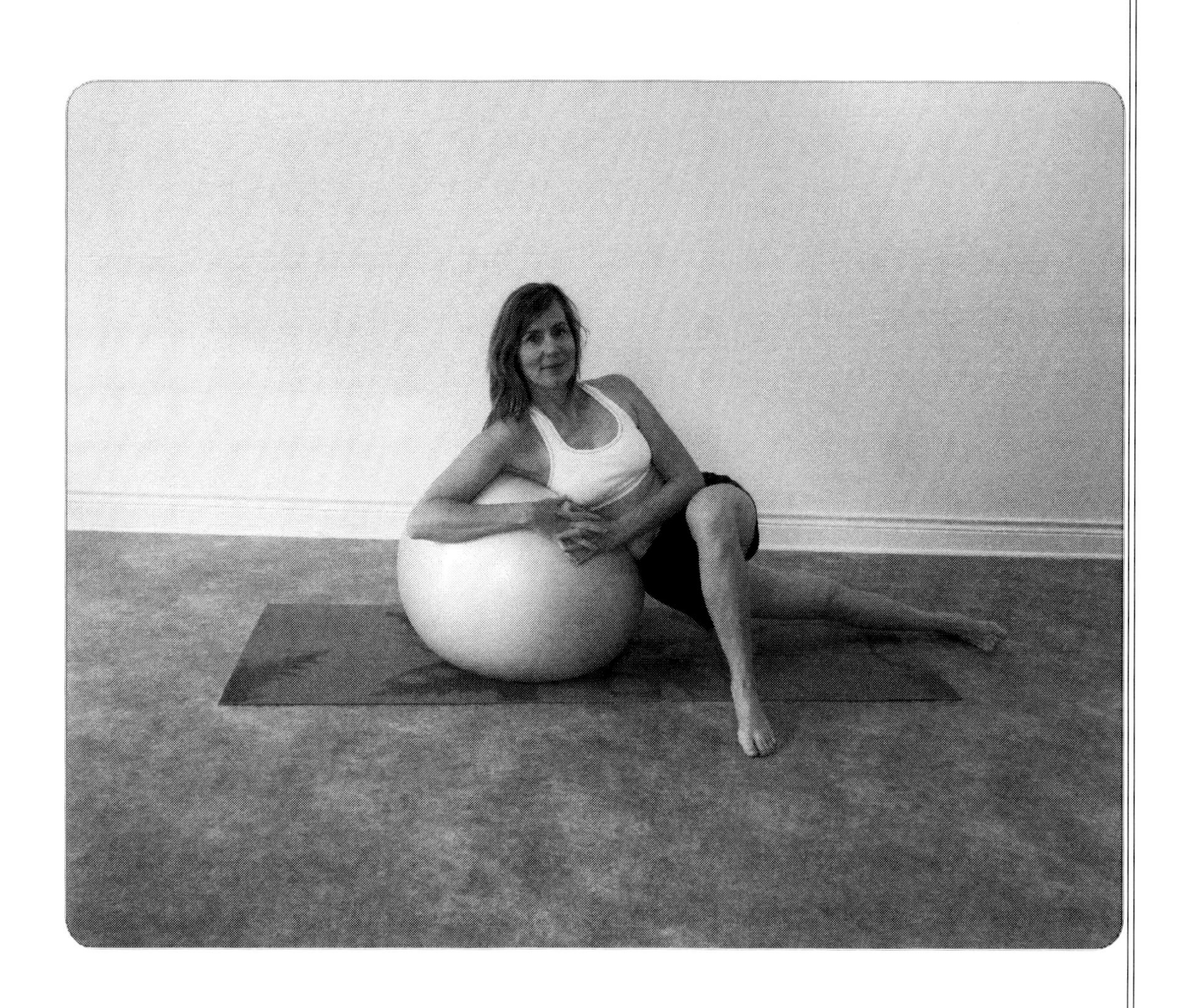

Client Education

Client education and compliance are crucial in restoring power, ease, and fluidity to the low back and pelvis. Our clients need and want our expertise for suggestions on self-care strategies such as sleep position, stretches, strengthening movements, and other self-care strategies.

In this section you'll find:

1. Suggestions for sleep position
2. Suggestions for self-care in the acute stage
3. Self-stretches for the iliopsoas, quadratus lumborum, and low back
4. Self-massage techniques with a MyoBall
5. Strengthening exercises
6. Movement suggestions

Once your client is out of the acute stage and in the recovery and maintenance stage she can keep her low back/pelvis contented and satisfied with a regular routine of stretching, Myoball self-massage and simple strength training movements. Begin with introducing self-stretches, the myoball self-massage, and gradually incorporate strength training exercises, beginning with Cobra pose.

Sleep Position

Sleep position is vital in resolving the perpetuating factors in low back/hip issues. One of the first questions you should ask a client is *"What position do you sleep in?"* Making that simple change can be profoundly valuable in decreasing your client's level of pain and the long-term outcome of your work.

Side-sleepers: Place a pillow between the knees as shown below. *Clients should avoid side-lying in a tight fetal position that excessively shortens the iliopsoas.*

Back sleepers: Place a pillow under the knees.

Stomach sleepers: Place a small, flat pillow or towel under the hips.

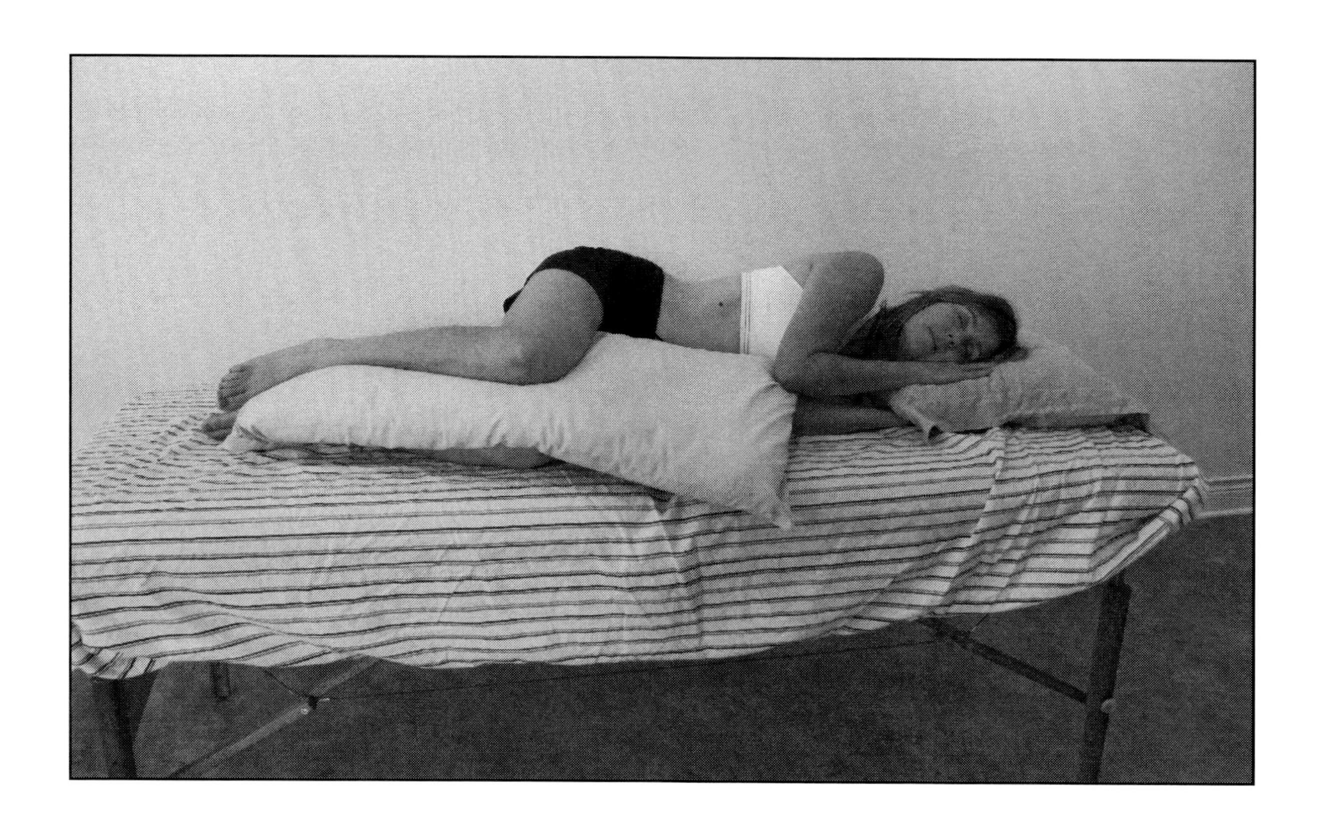

If your client is in the acute pain stage, the following four poses are the best self-care strategies to start with. They unload the spine and place the low back/pelvis in a neutral position. If any of these poses cause pain, either modify the pose till it feels right or discontinue the pose.

1. Legs Over the Chair/Ottoman (this pose can be done lying on an ice pack):

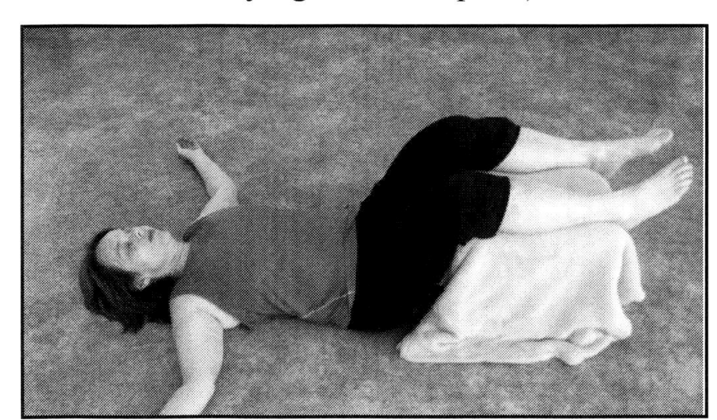

- Lie on your back.
- Drape your legs over a chair, ottoman, or any piece of furniture that is not too high.
- Legs should be hip distance apart, knees and ankles aligned with each other.
- Allow the spine, neck, jaw, and shoulders to lengthen and relax into the floor.
- Allow the arms to rest comfortably by your side or on your belly.
- Feel the support of stable and solid Mother Earth.
- Breathe deeply and relax.

2. Constructive Rest Position (this pose can be done lying on an ice pack):

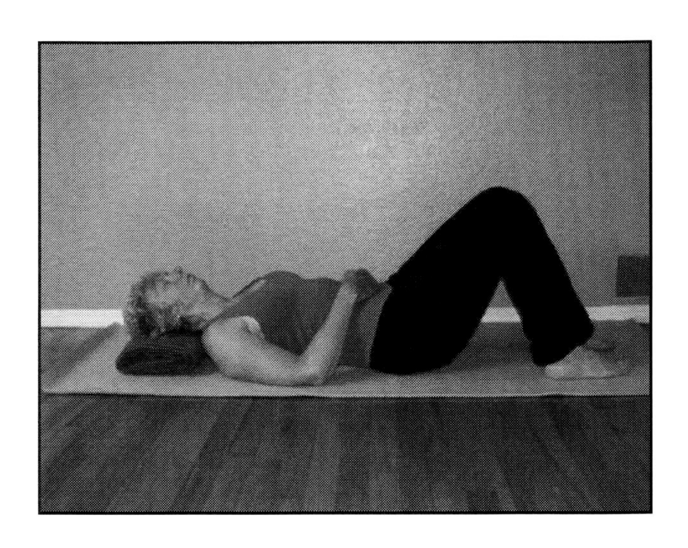

- Lie on your back.
- Bend your knees and put your feet flat on the floor.
- Legs should be hip distance apart, knees and ankles aligned with each other.
- Allow the spine, neck, jaw and shoulders to lengthen and relax into the floor.
- Allow the arms to rest comfortably by your side or on your belly.
- Feel the support of stable and solid Mother Earth.
- Breathe deeply and relax.

You can add gentle side-to-side rocking of the legs for additional release if it does not cause any pain.

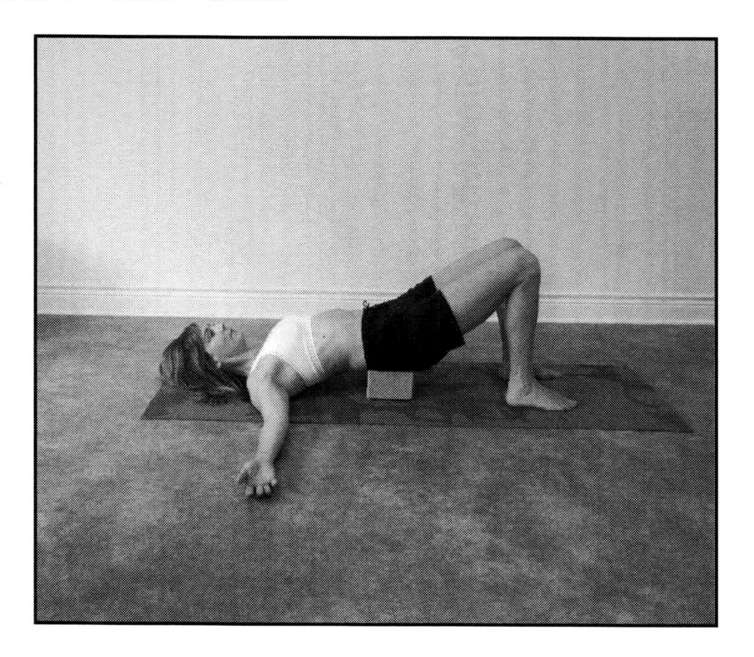

3. Low back/sacrum alignment with a yoga block:
This is a gentle stretch for the low back that also helps with lumbar/sacral alignment:

- Start with the body in neutral position: knees bent and feet on the floor.
- Slide a yoga block under the sacrum and position it where it feels the most comfortable.
- Position the arms in a T shape, with-palms up for a gentle opening through the chest.
- Enjoy and hold for as long as you like.

4. Legs Up the Wall (this pose can be done lying on an ice pack). Getting into this pose can be painful in the acute stage so approach with caution.

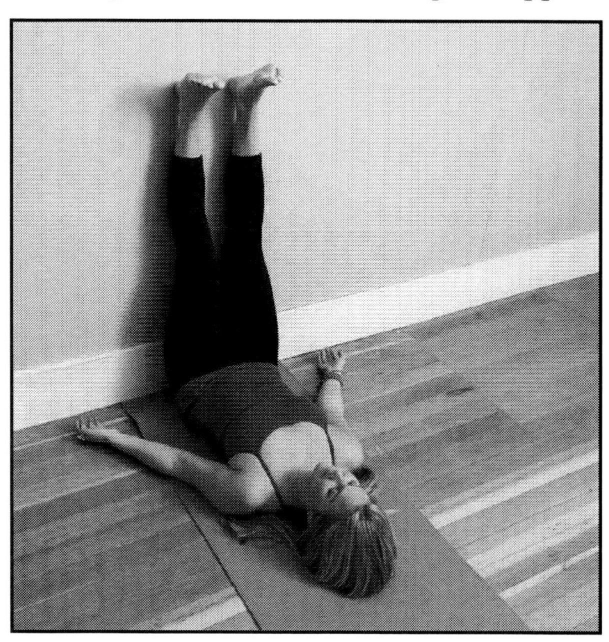

- Sit on the floor with your right side touching the wall.
- Gently turn your body and bring your legs up onto the wall. Use your hands for balance as you shift your weight. Lower your back to the floor and lie down.
- Shift your weight from side-to-side and scoot your buttocks close to the wall.
- Legs should be hip distance apart, knees and ankles aligned with each other.
- Allow the spine, neck, jaw, and shoulders to lengthen and relax into the floor.
- Allow the arms to rest comfortably by your side or on your belly.
- Feel the support of stable and solid Mother Earth.
- Breathe deeply and relax.

To release, slowly push yourself away from the wall and slide your legs down to the right side. Use your hands to help press yourself back up into a seated position.

Iliopsoas/Thigh Flexor Self-Stretches

The most common way to stretch all the hip flexors is through a lunge position, with the knee either on or off the floor. You'll see both variations and also a version of this stretch using an exercise ball.

Since there are nine thigh flexors, it's critical that all of them have an opportunity to be stretched. In addition to the usual version with the thigh in neutral, we'll add variations that include internally and externally rotating the thigh, which stretches the lateral and medial thigh flexors — similar to the assisted table stretches.

Kneeling Iliopsoas/Thigh Flexor Stretch: This is a good beginning stretch for locked short thigh flexors.

Step One: Kneel on left knee, with toes down, and place right foot flat on the floor in front of you, knee bent and aligned with ankle. Place hands on right thigh.

Step Two: Press hips forward until you feel a stretch in the front of your left thigh. Hold each position shown below for 15-30 seconds, then switch sides.

For more intensity, extend arms overhead, with elbows close to head and palms facing each other, and slightly arch your back while keeping your chin parallel to the ground.

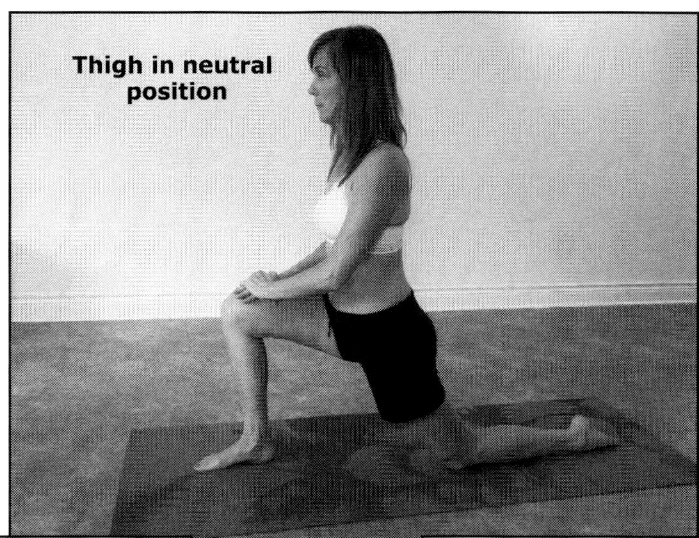

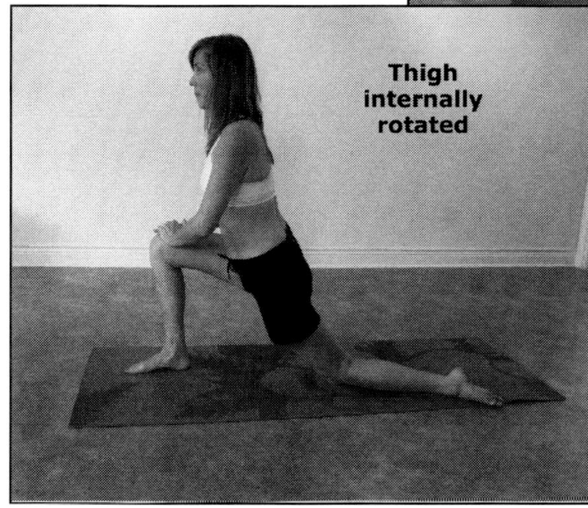

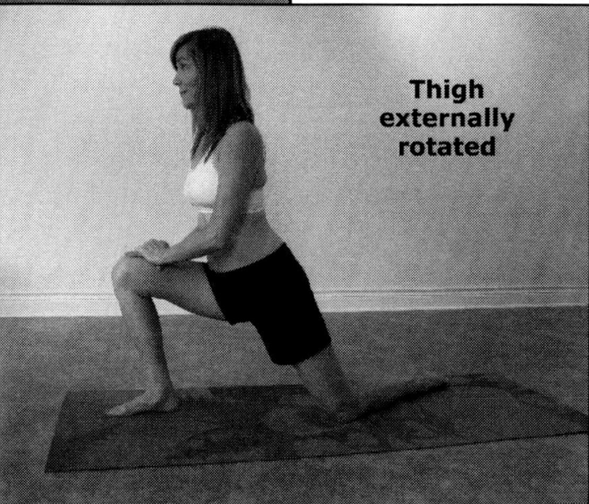

Lunging Iliopsoas/Thigh Flexor Stretch: This is a more intense stretch for locked short thigh flexors.

Step forward into a lunge far enough so that you have to bend your front leg, but not so far so that you can't keep the ball of your opposite foot on the ground. Sink down into the lunge, feeling the pull on your back quad and calf. Make sure the knee is aligned with the ankle.

The spine is in neutral and your pelvis is slightly tucked under your body. Hold each position shown below for 15-30 seconds, then release. Repeat with the opposite leg.

For more intensity, extend arms overhead, with elbows close to head and palms facing each other, and slightly arch your back while keeping your chin parallel to the ground.

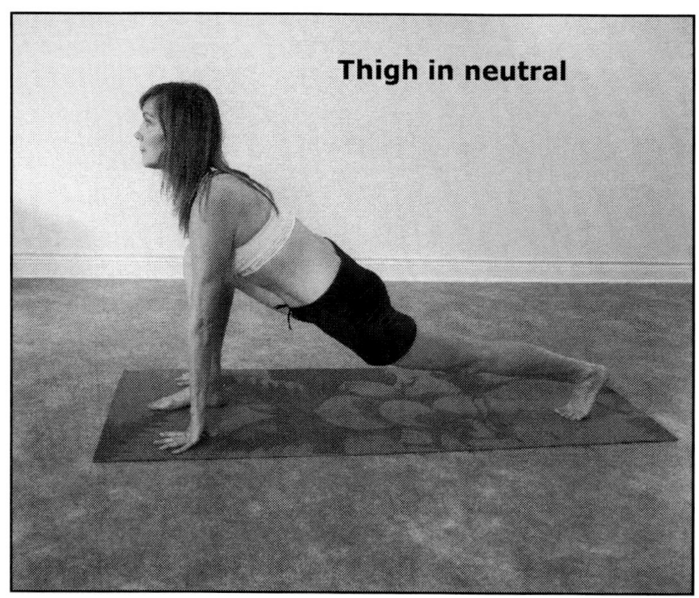
Thigh in neutral

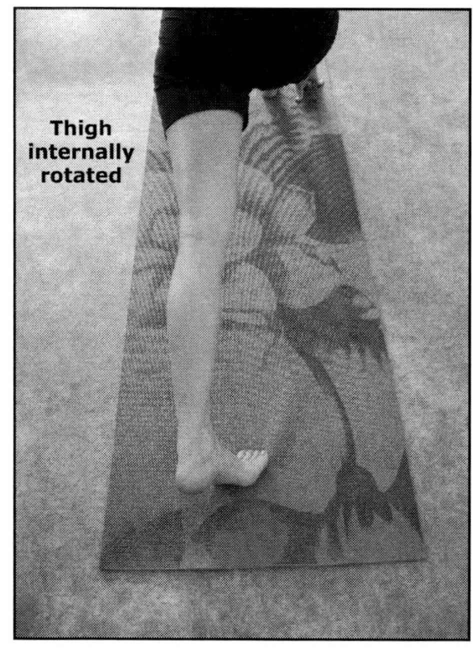
Thigh internally rotated

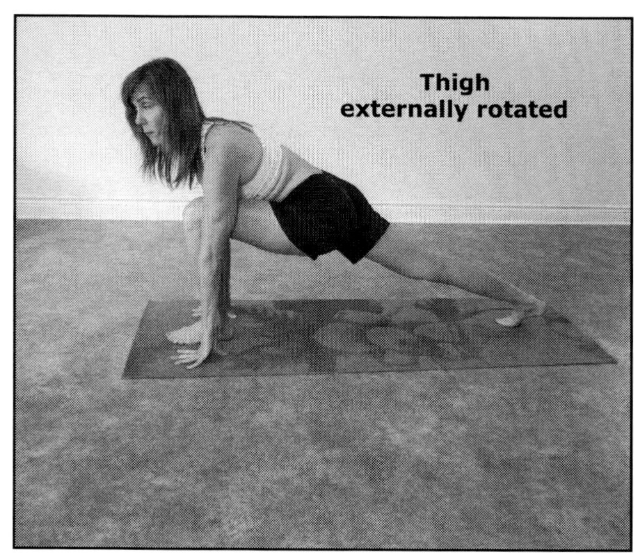
Thigh externally rotated

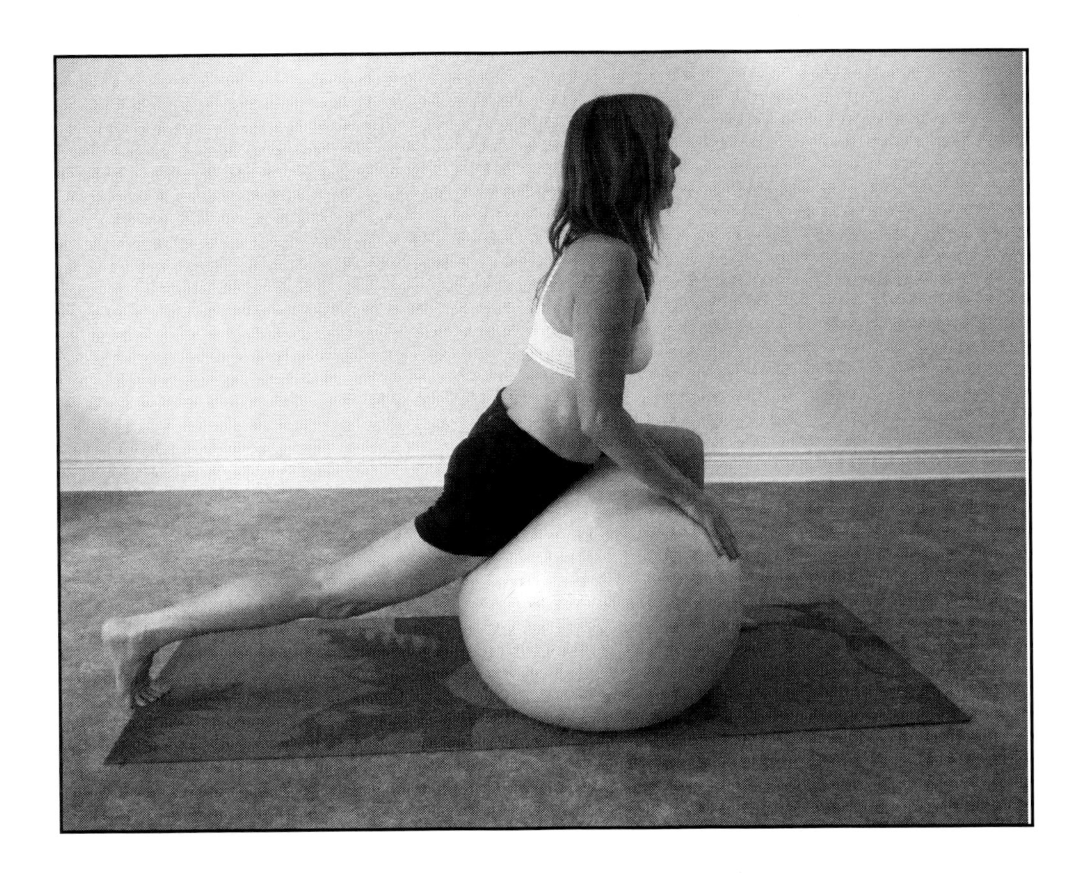

Lunging Iliopsoas/Thigh Flexor Stretch with Exercise Ball: This the same stretch as on the previous page with the added support of an exercise ball.

The photo below shows the *right* quadratus lumborum being stretched.

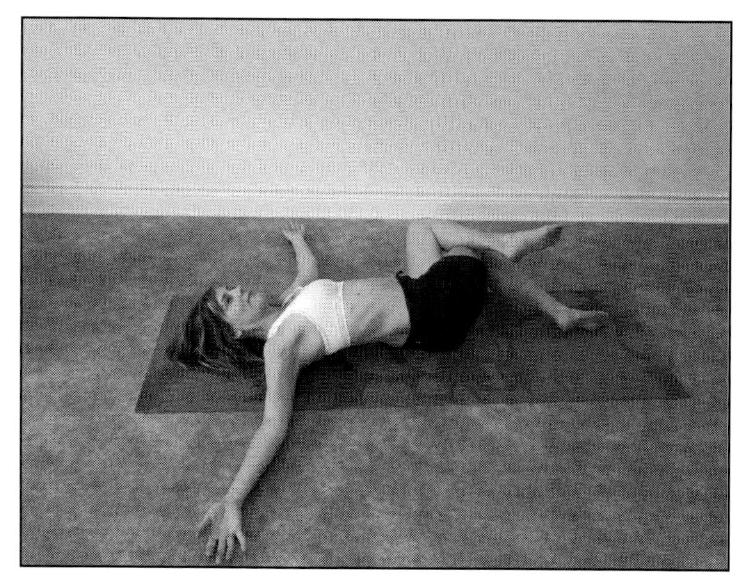

Cross the left knee (make sure it's the knee, not the ankle) over the right and use your left leg to pull your right leg across and towards the floor. It's not important that the right knee reaches the floor — stretch within your limits.

Notice the placement of the arms. They must be above the ribs to properly stretch the quadratus lumborum since it attaches at the 12th rib.

To increase the stretch in the quadratus lumborum, increase the thigh flexion in the side being stretched. Less thigh flexion puts more stretch on the gluteus medius and minimus, tensor fascia latae and iliotibial band.

Hold for 15-30 seconds and repeat on other side.

QL stretch with Exercise Ball:

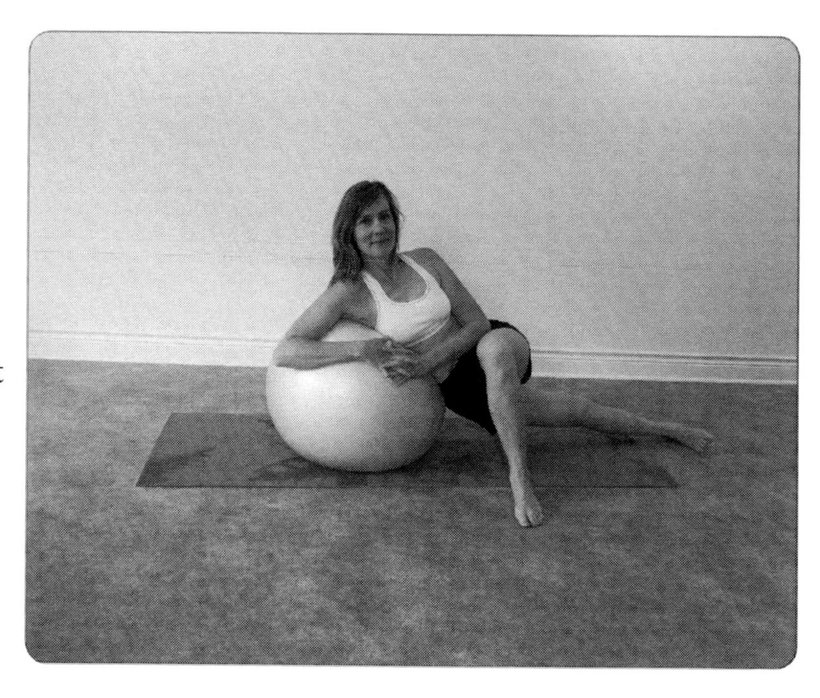

The photo at right shows the *right* quadratus lumborum being stretched. This is a wonderful stretch that has the added support of an exercise ball.

Step One: Kneel on the floor next to the ball. Lean the side being stretched on the ball.

Step Two: Cross the top leg over the bottom leg.

Step Three: Press into the top foot and lift the hips off the floor.

Hold for 15-30 seconds and repeat on other side.

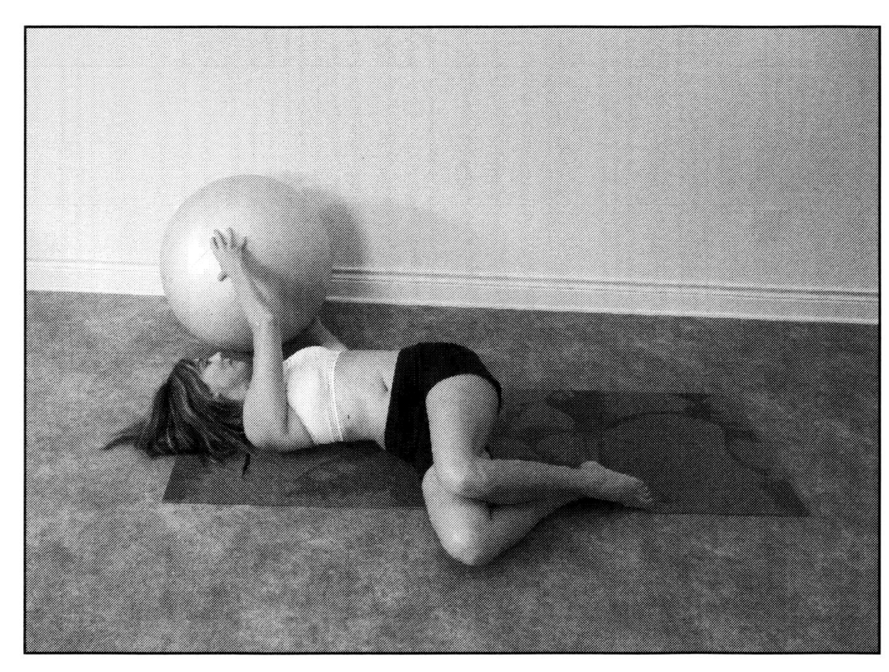

This yummy spinal twist stretch is simple and sweet!

Step One: Start with the body in neutral position – knees bent, feet on the floor, holding an exercise ball.

Step Two: Let the knees comfortably fall to the right as you let the ball fall the left.

Step Three: Enjoy and hold for 15-30 seconds. Repeat on the other side.

This delicious stretch can also be done without a ball as shown below.

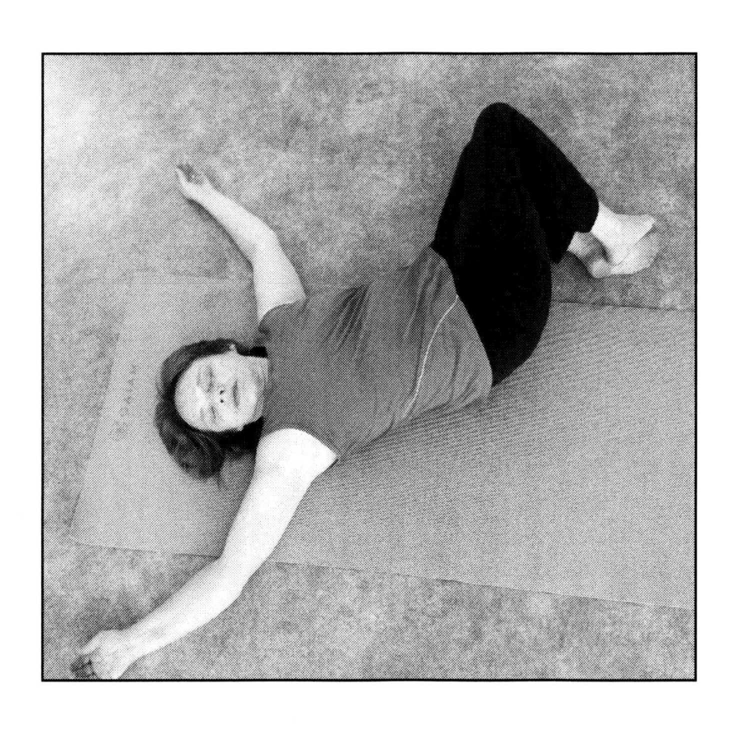

More Self-Stretches for the Low Back

Hugging one or both knees into the torso is a staple of good low back self-care as shown in the top two photos. This stretch gently lengthens tissue while the floor provides a supporting surface, reminding us that our stable and strong Mother Earth "has our back."

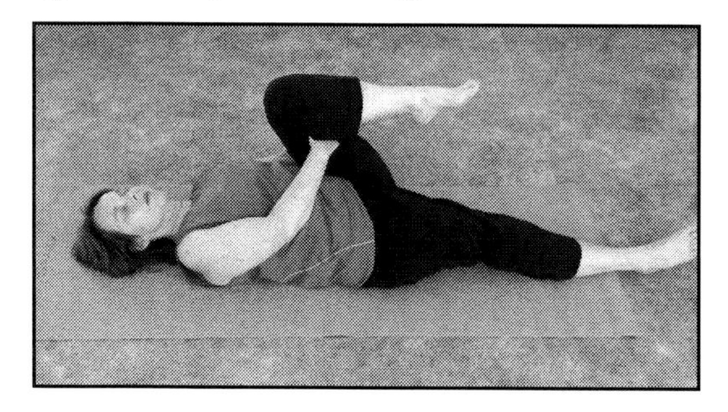

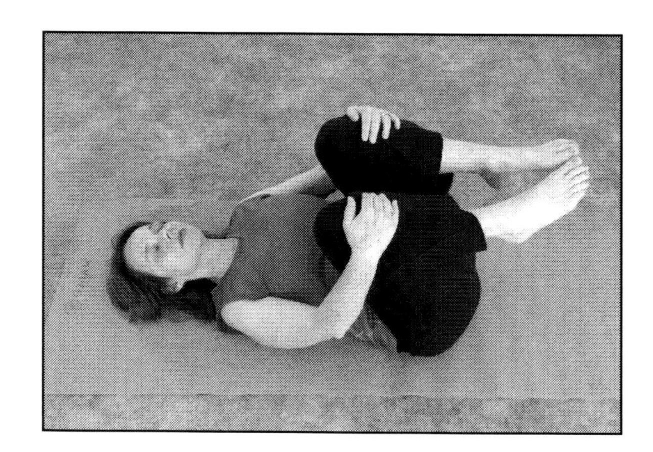

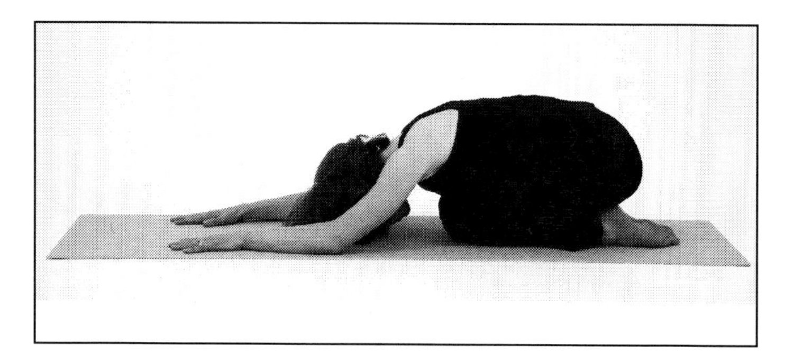

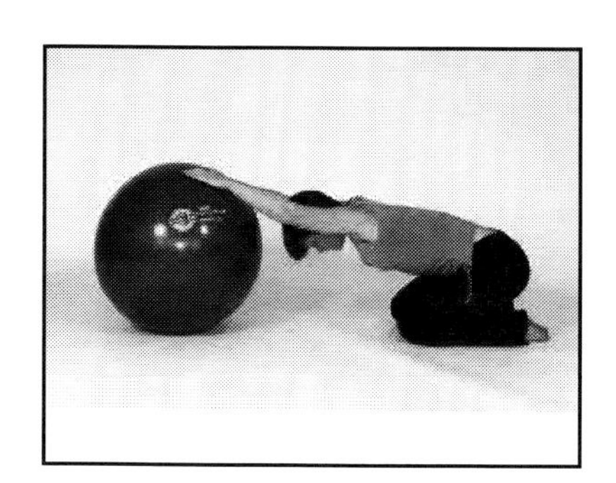

Pose of child is a deeply nurturing stretch that is especially good for an anteriorly tilted pelvis as shown above:

Step One: Begin kneeling on your mat or floor with your butt on your heels.

Step Two: With your toes together, open your knees to at least hip distance apart.

Step Three: Lean forward and drape your body over your thighs so that your forehead rests on the floor or a pillow.

Step Four: Reach your arms out in front of you. Alternately, you can leave your arms along your sides. Try both and see which feels best to you.

TIP: A towel or pillow on top of the calves helps to reduce knee strain. A towel or pillow on top of the thighs creates space for a large girth, facilitating deep breathing.

This stretch can also be done with a ball as shown above right.

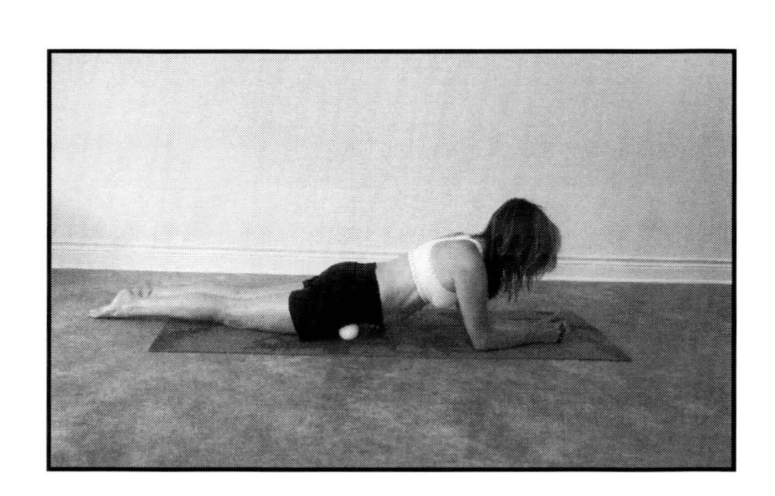

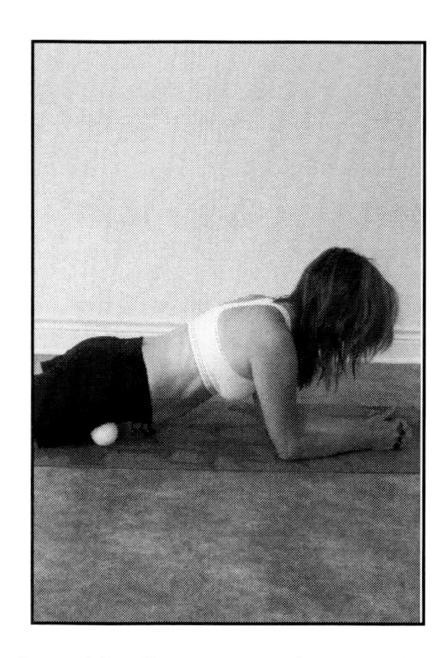

Place a MyoBall or tennis ball anywhere on the secondary hip flexors as shown above. Gently apply pressure by slowly lowering the body weight. Hold until you feel a release.

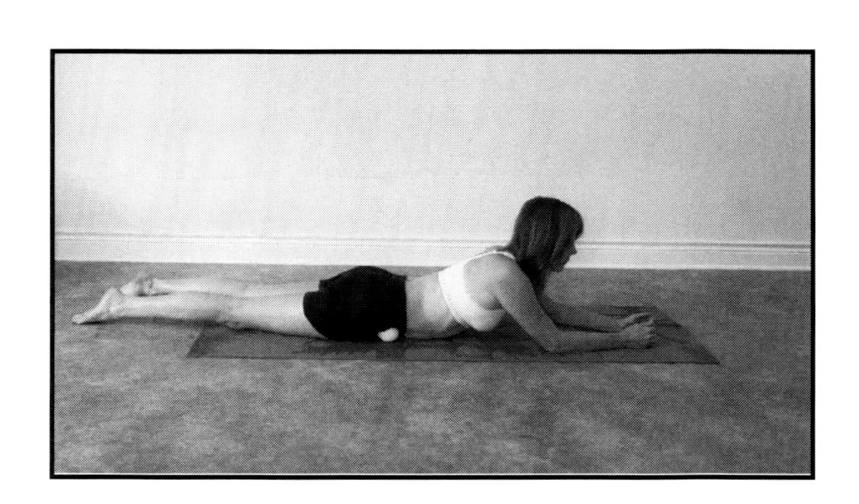

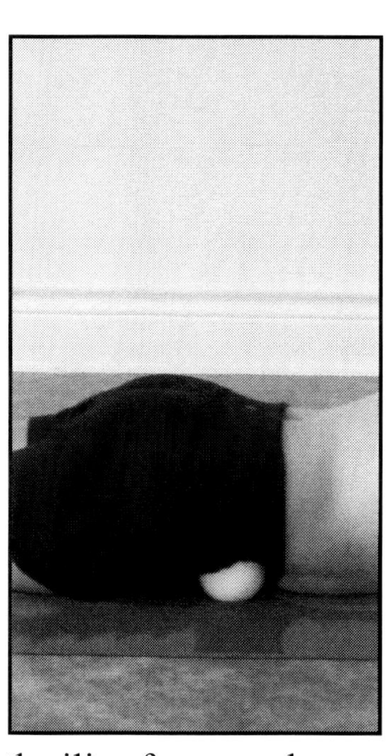

Place a MyoBall or tennis ball medial to the iliac crest in the iliac fossa as shown above. Gently apply pressure by slowly lowering the body weight. Hold until you feel a release.

Strength Training Exercises for the Low Back/Core

One of the most effective and simple exercises for strengthening the low back and core is the Cobra pose.

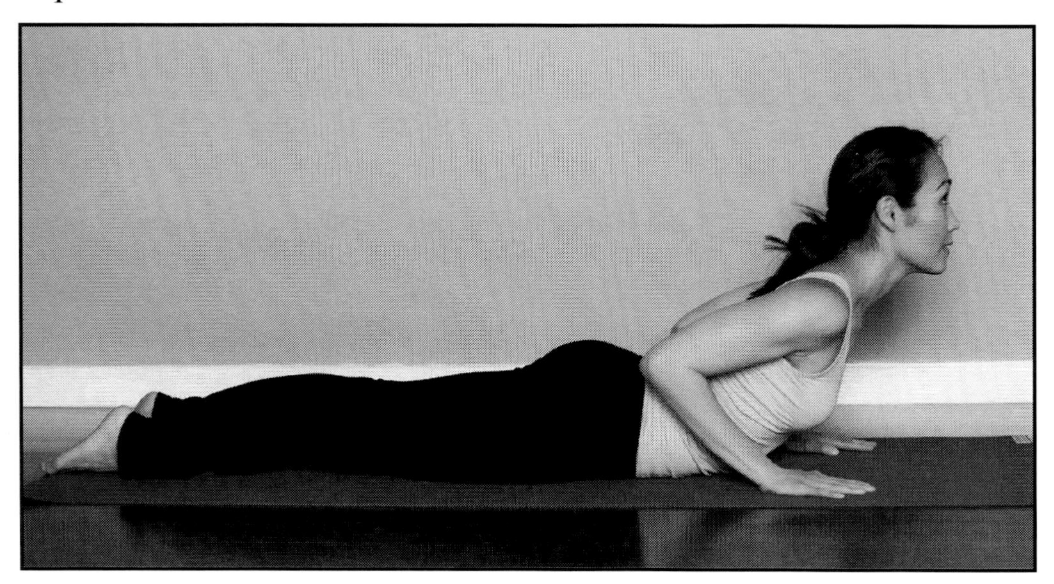

This easy exercise can do wonders to fortify and restore tone to weak, flaccid low back muscles.

Step One: Lie prone on the floor. Stretch your legs back, tops of the feet on the floor. Spread your hands on the floor under your shoulders. Hug the elbows into your body. Allow the shoulder blades to slide toward the low back.

Step Two: Slowly lift the sternum off the floor but avoid pushing the front ribs forward, which only hardens the lower back. Lift only to the height at which you can maintain a connection through your pubic bone to your legs. Distribute the backbend evenly throughout the entire spine. Gently press the tailbone toward the pubic bone and lift the pubic bone toward the navel. The buttocks stay loose.

Hold the pose anywhere from 15-30 seconds, breathing easily. Release back to the floor with an exhalation.

You can modify this pose for less intensity by placing your forearms on the floor rather than the palms. Following up with a gentle back stretch is a good idea, to keep muscles in balance. Child's pose is an ideal follow-up to the Cobra.

People with facet joint problems, for example, spondylolisthesis, should approach cobra pose cautiously, if at all. Facet joint problems tend to become irritated when the spine is arched. Ask your doctor or physical therapist if this pose is okay for your condition.

If you are in acute pain, the cobra pose should not be attempted. Otherwise, listen carefully to your pain and let it guide you as to how far you go with the pose.

Sit-backs and planks are more advanced exercises that should be done when the client has experienced a significant reduction in pain and is ready to build more core strength. Many people have what I call "gym abs" meaning they have strong concentric strength from doing hundreds of crunches. They might look good but still have a weak core. I recommend developing eccentric and isometric strength to acquire core stability and functional movement. Sit-backs are good for developing eccentric strength, and planks are great for developing isometric strength.

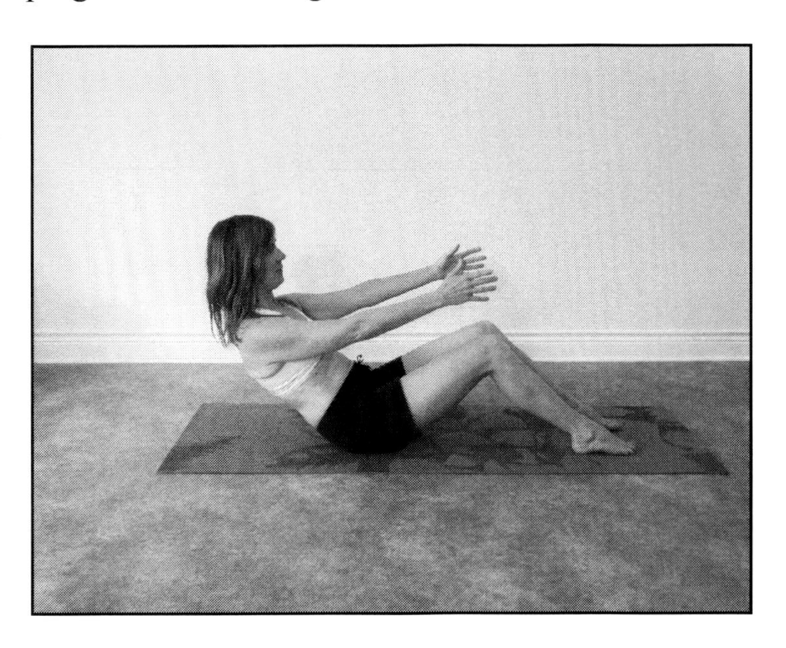

Sit-Backs:

Step One: Sit with your knees bent and feet firmly planted on the floor, ankles and knees aligned. This is neutral position. Arms can be outstretched in front or crossed over the chest.

Step Two: Curl the pelvis under.

Step Three: On an exhale, slowly roll back as far as comfortable.

Step Four: Hold for 15 seconds.

Step Five: On an inhale, return to neutral position.

Step Six: Repeat until the abdominals fatigue.

Step Seven: Follow with a low back stretch of your choice such as Pose of child or hugging both knees into the torso.

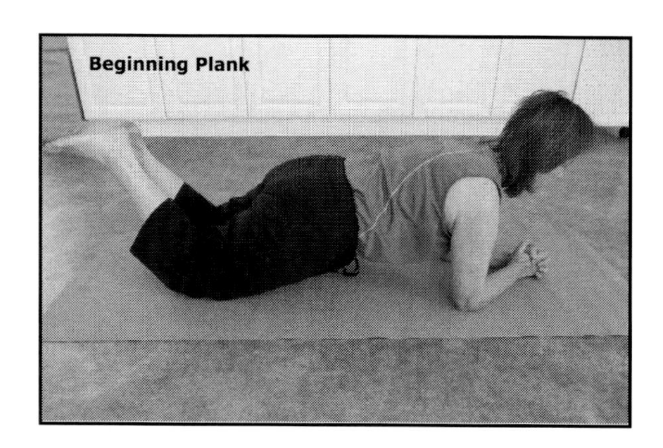

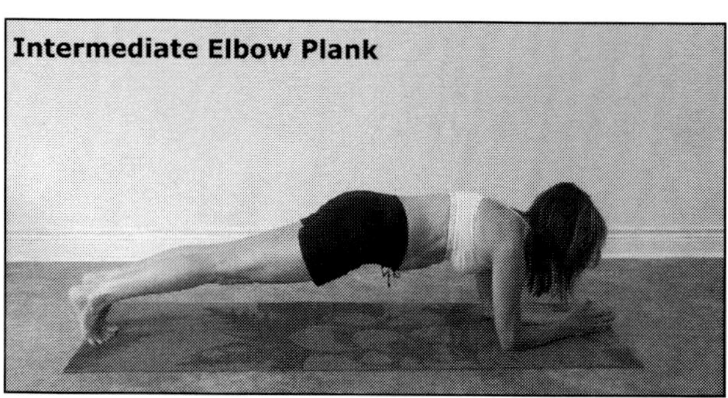

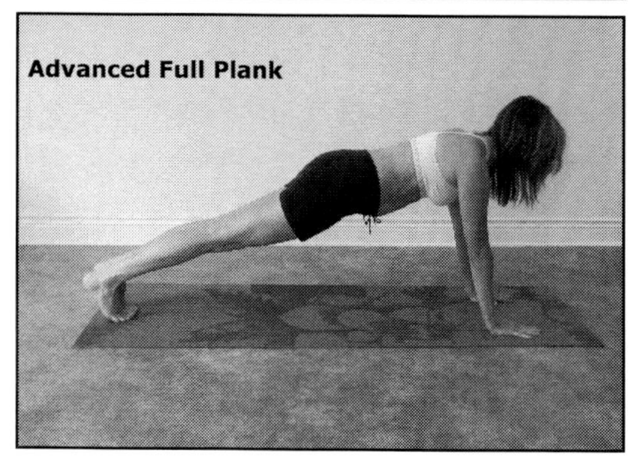

Planks: According to the American Council on Exercise, the plank exercise is one of the top ten abdominal exercises. But bad form can hurt the shoulders and back. The most common mistakes are collapsing at the lower back and shoulders, and, having the arms in what I call the "bull dog" position with the shoulders internally rotated, scapulae protracted and elbows bent. The directions below are for both the beginner and advanced versions. Start with the beginner version, which can also be done with the knees on the floor for less intensity.

Step One: Kneel on the floor or mat. Place your elbows or arms directly beneath your shoulders – joints in one line (like a skyscraper). Weight should be transferred through the center of the joints. The hands may be flexed into a fist or relaxed.

Step Two: Retract the scapulae and slide the shoulders away from the ears. Externally rotate the shoulder joints by moving the triceps toward one another.

Step Three: The spine should be lengthened in equal opposite directions. Lift your head away from your shoulders, lengthening your neck while simultaneously reaching your tailbone in the other direction. Do not round the spine or hyperextend the neck. Maintain this long spine throughout the entire duration.

Step Three: Begin by holding the plank for 10-15 seconds, gradually increasing your time by adding 5-10 seconds as you gain strength. Follow with a low back stretch of your choice.

A unique benefit of the exercise or stability ball stems from the ability to position the body with proper alignment and simultaneously challenge a muscle or group of muscles. Maintaining proper alignment on the ball stimulates the body's natural motor reflexes and encourages the body to react as a whole, integrated unit. In other words, the ball challenges the whole body to participate in order to maintain correct posture and balance, and to perform the dynamic movement. The Supine Bridge below is an outstanding exercise for strength training the core.

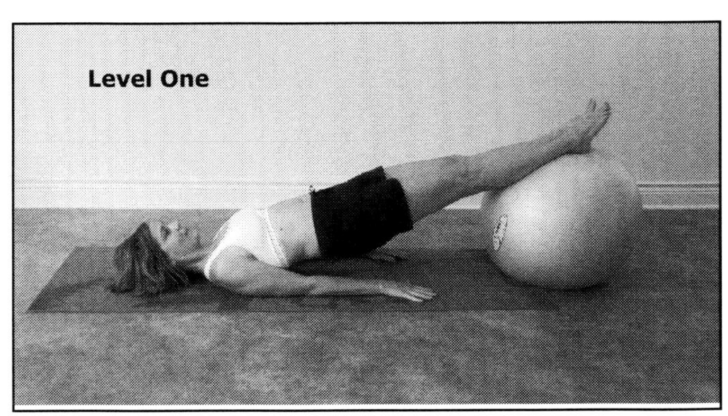

Supine Bridge With Exercise Ball:
Step One: Lying supine with heels, ankles, and lower legs hip width apart on the ball.

Step Two: Curl the pelvis under, then slowly lift the pelvis off the floor. Your arms are on the floor by your side in a comfortable position. Keep the gluteus maximus relaxed. Let the core do the work. Hold for 15-30 seconds.

Step Three: To come out, curl the pelvis under and lower the spine vertebrae by vertebrae.

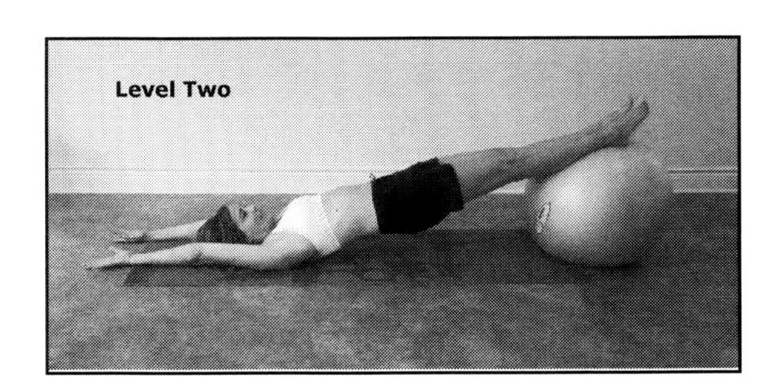

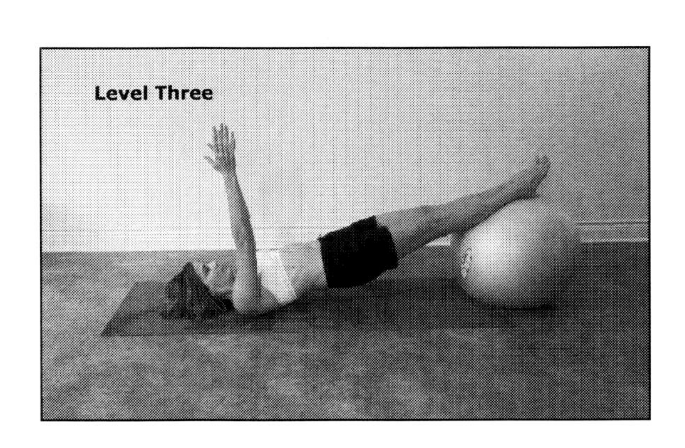

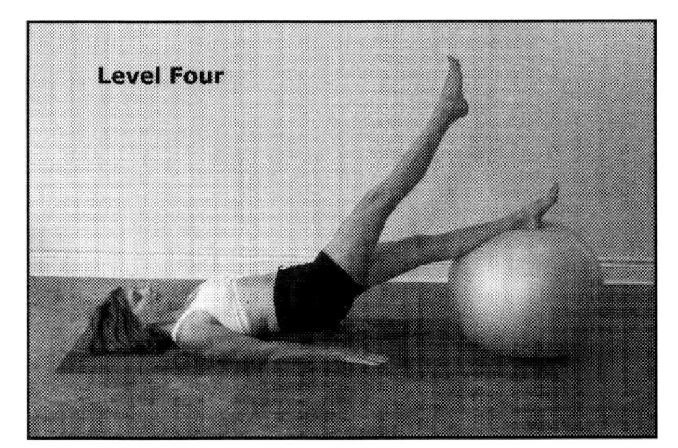

One of the great things about exercise balls is that a simple change of arm position totally changes the difficulty of an exercise. After gaining mastery of Level One, challenge your balance and coordination by changing your arm position as shown in Levels Two and Three. Once you've mastered those variations, try the ultimate version of this exercise by lifting one leg off the ball!

Movement Suggestions

In order for the pelvis to hang freely a supple iliopsoas is necessary and low back strength and flexibility can be developed through moving the pelvis in novel and unusual ways.

Movement allows us to feel alive, vital, and passionate about life. When we move in a variety of ways, different parts of our nervous system are stimulated, giving us a fresh sense of ourselves, a fresh identity. Below are some movement suggestions that I've used myself for many years, taught to students and clients from age five to ninety five. These movements encourage a new and happy sense of movement. Doing these movement to your favorite music is highly recommended!

1. Pelvic tilts are a beautiful and easy exercise for increasing proprioception throughout the low back and pelvis. The best way to do them without using incorrect muscular effort is to imagine the pubic bone moving toward and away from the belly button. When we initiate moving from our bones, the correct and most efficient neuromuscular pathways are created. I suggest starting with small pelvic tilts (micro-movements) then slowly increasing the range of movement.

2. As you stand, circle your hips around an imaginary hula hoop. Feel your pelvis touching the entire rim of the hoop as you circle your hips to release the low back and increase pelvic range of motion. Hip circles transmit and conduct blocked energy from the iliopsoas and quadratus lumborum down through our lower body, rejuvenating our second chakra.

3. Imagine there's a big paint brush extending from your belly button. Pick your favorite color and write your first and last name with the paint brush. Then, move the paint brush to your tail bone and write your first and last name with the paint brush. Cross your T's and dot your I's!

4. Standing pelvic tilts using a wall: Stand facing a wall and place your palms, shoulder height, on the wall. Lift your heels slightly off the floor. Swing the pelvis toward and away from the wall about ten times. This exercise helps to discharge excess energy and tension in the pelvis/low back and move it down the legs and out the feet.

Bibliography

Anderson, Bob: Stretching; Shelter Publications; 2010.
Bainbridge-Cohen, Bonnie: Sensing, Feeling, and Action; Contact Editions; 1993.
Berceli, David; Trauma Releasing Exercises; DVD, 2004.
Berceli, David & Koch, Liz: The Iliopsoas Muscle Parts One and Two; Massage Magazine; May/June 2005.
Clay, James H. & Pounds, David M: Basic Clinical Massage Therapy: Integrating Anatomy and Treatment; Lippincott Williams & Wilkins, 2003.
Carrico, Maria: Yoga Basics; Henry Holt and Compnay; 1997.
Davies, Clair: The Trigger Point Therapy Workbook; New Harbinger Publications, Inc., 2001.
Dychtwald, Ken: BodyMind; Tarcher Putman; 1977.
Johnson, Don Hanlon: Bone, Breath and Gesture; North Atlantic Books, 1995.
Earls, James, Myers, Thomas: Fascial Release for Structural Balance; North Atlantic Books; 2010.
Hamill, Joseph & Knutzen, Kathleen: Biomechanical Basis of Human Movement, Lippincott, Williams & Williams, 1995.
Hartley, Linda: Wisdom of the Body Moving; North Atlantic Books, 1995.
Juan, Dean: Job's Body; Station Hill Press; 1987.
Kent, Howard: Yoga Made Easy; Quarto Publishing; 1993.
Koch, Liz; Trauma Recovery Protocol; Massage & Bodywork, December/January 2004.
Lamb, Peggy: Stretch Your Clients: The Bodyworker's Guide to Client Table Stretches; Massage Publications; 2012.
Lowe, Whitney: Functional Assessment in Massage Therapy, 2nd edition, Pacific Orthopedic Massage, 1995.
Lowen, Alexander, Lowen, Leslie, Skalecki Walter: The Way to Vibrant Health: A Manual of Bioenergetic Exercises; Bioenergetics Press; 2003.
Lowen, Alexander: Bioenergetics: The Revolutionary Therapy That Uses the Language of the Body to Heal the Problems of the Mind; Bioenergetics Press; 1994.
Myers, Thomas: The Opinionated Psoas - Parts 1-4; Massage and Bodywork; 2001.
Myers, Thomas: Anatomy Trains; Elsevier; 2008.
Newton, Don: Clinical Pathology for the Professional Bodyworker, Simran Publications, 1998.
Sacks, Oliver: A Leg to Stand On; HarperCollins; 1984.
Schultz, R. Louis & Feitis, Rosemary: The Endless Web, North Atlantic Books, 1996.
Sweigard, Lulu: Human Movement Potential: Its Ideokinetic Facilitation; Harper and Row, 1974.
Todd, Mabel: The Thinking Body; Paul Hoeber, Inc, 1937.
Travell, Janet & Simons, David: Myofascial Pain and Dysfunction - The Trigger Point Manual, Volumes 1 & 2, William & Wilkins, 1983.

Index